# Obstetrics and Gynaecology in Tudor and Stuart England

Audrey Eccles

The Kent State University Press

Published in the United States of America by
The Kent State University Press, Kent, Ohio 44242

**Library of Congress Cataloging in Publication Data**

Eccles, Audrey.
Obstetrics and gynaecology in Tudor and Stuart England
1. Obstetrics – England – History – 16th century.
2. Obstetrics – England – History – 17th century.
3. Gynecology – England – History – 16th century.
4. Gynecology – England – History – 17th century.
I. Title. (DNLM: 1. Gynecology –History – England.
2. History of Medicine, 16th century – England.
3. History of Medicine, 17th century – England.
4. Obstetrics – History – England. WQ 11 FE5 E170)
RG518.G7E25 1982 618'.00942 81-19374

ISBN 0-87338-270-6 AACR2

Printed and bound in Great Britain

# Contents

# Preface

Historians have paid much attention to the origin of ideas about generation, anatomy and physiology in ancient times, and to the discovery of new facts and the introduction of new methods during the Renaissance and since. This interest in discovery and development has, however, overshadowed investigations into the time new scientific ideas took to gain general acceptance, and into the persistence of older ideas at more popular levels.

In this book I propose to examine the rise of new ideas in obstetrics and the fall of old ones in the literature meant for practitioners. This ranges from translations of the work of important scientists, to potboilers written by people with very little knowledge of midwifery for people with even less. The public was evidently fascinated by the subject and it tended to be the more popular and less scientific texts which were most frequently reprinted.

The period I shall discuss extends from 1540, when *The birth of mankind* was first published, to about 1740, by which date advancing knowledge had brought about far-reaching changes in midwifery, both as a scientifically-based skill, and as a social phenomenon.

The rise of the man-midwife is a complex subject which I hope to explore in detail in a future book, but the changes in knowledge and practice described in this book were an essential forerunner to that departure from the custom of centuries. Science provided the impetus and the rationale for a new view of obstetrics and of the persons practising it.

It is notoriously difficult to write about the beliefs and customs of ordinary people, since they rarely leave much documentary record. But much incidental information can be found about traditions and beliefs in these textbooks, and it is on this material that I chiefly base my statements about popular thought and practice. Archival evidence from diaries, letters etc. suggests that this is not an unreasonable assumption, but it would be interesting to have considerably more such material brought to light in order to test the reliability of the statements in the printed works.

# Acknowledgements

In the course of fifteen years' work on the early English midwiferies and related topics I have accumulated more debts of honour than I can hope to mention. I should like however to express my gratitude for the support of my husband and family, and to thank the following people for particular assistance: Miss Sheila MacPherson, Deputy County Archivist, Cumbria and Mr David Cook, Medical Sub-librarian, Manchester University, have both afforded me exceptional research facilities without which this work would have been much more difficult to complete. I am much indebted over many years to Mr Eric Freeman of the Wellcome Library and his staff. Mr Richard Samways of the Greater London Record Office has unstintingly provided hospitality and encouragement on my frequent visits to London libraries. Dr Chris Land FRCOG has generously explained many points in obstetrics, especially in interpreting the Willughby cases. Dr Charles Webster, Reader in the History of Medicine at the Wellcome Unit, Oxford, kindly read the first four chapters in manuscript, and the notes on blood-letting are largely a result of his comments, the notes on the nitro-aerial particles entirely so. I am also grateful to many searchers at the record office, Kendal, in the years I was an archivist there, and to various members of the Society for the Social History of Medicine, especially to Mr Adrian Wilson, for helpful suggestions, criticisms and references. My thanks also go to Mr Richard Samways for compiling the index.

*Chapter One*

# English Obstetrical Textbooks Before 1740

Not much is known about the practice of obstetrics in the mediaeval period, although it is possible to form an idea of the theory from extant manuscripts. No doubt in some cases theory approximated to practice, but in others, especially among the unlettered classes, midwifery was a traditional women's business, about the actual conduct of which it is unlikely much can now be discovered.

The standard mediaeval text on obstetrics was a Latin work generally called *Trotula*, after the name of its author. It was this book that Chaucer's doctor of physic used, and the name at least seems to have been familiar to his audience. Trotula is said to have been a female doctor in the eleventh century at the then prestigious medical school of Salerno, and in her book claims to have specialised in women's diseases out of sympathy for women too modest to consult male doctors about gynaecological problems.[1] Some of the details in her book show that if theory and practice agreed at all, the mediaeval woman may have fared better in some respects than her Tudor and Stuart counterpart.

The book is, for the period, highly scientific in tone, and recommends sensible practices such as the suture of perineal tears, and the treatment of prolapse by manual reduction, bed rest and a low residue diet. It is not helpful, however, in cases of abnormal births, which are mainly dealt with by medicines. The anatomy, physiology and therapy of the book generally, is firmly in the tradition of humoral medicine.

Manuscript translations of *Libri Trotuli* began to appear in English in the late fourteenth and fifteenth centuries, several of which are still extant.[2] However, the advent of printing made it possible to bring mediaeval works including those on midwifery, thought to be of current interest, to a far wider public despite a good deal of opposition on moral grounds.[3] The earliest English textbook for midwives in print was *The birth of mankind*. First published in 1540, it was translated by Richard Jonas from *De partu hominis*, which itself was a translation made in 1532 by Christian Egenolph from a German original.

This German original, *Der swangern Frauwen und Hebammen Roszgarten*, was published in 1513 by Eucharius Rösslin, state physician of Worms and Frankfurt-am-Main, for the instruction of the official town midwives.

Evidently *The birth of mankind* filled a need, for in 1545 it was revised and reissued under the same title by Thomas Raynald. Raynald styled himself 'physician', but it is doubtful if he had any practical experience of midwifery himself. He claimed that the book had already been of much use at labours, gentlewomen having taken to visiting confinements 'carienge with them this booke in theyr handes, and causynge suche part of it as doth cheifly concerne the same pourpose, to be red before the mydwife, and the rest of the wemen then beyng present', with such good effect that right-minded women were glad 'to here the booke red by sum other, or els (such as could) to read it the*m* selfes'.[4] *The birth of mankind* ran into thirteen editions, the last in 1654, before it was finally superseded.[5]

There were also more popularly written texts aimed at a less-specialised public, which maintained their popularity at this level long past the period with which we are concerned. Quite when and where *Aristotle's complete masterpiece*, *Aristotle's experienced midwife*, and *Aristotle's last legacy* originated is obscure. The earliest edition of the experienced midwife in the British library is dated 1700, and signed W. S. (possibly William Salmon, a prolific writer of medical books) but the contents are certainly derived from much older works. There is a copy of the masterpiece dated 1694, and of the last legacy dated 1690. They were reissued frequently, and the masterpiece had reached 26 editions by the middle of the eighteenth century, the experienced midwife ten.[6] They are rare nowadays, and were, like many ephemera, clearly read to pieces and thrown away, not cherished as valuable textbooks.

Although Paré's work on obstetrics appeared in the original French in 1549 it was not translated into English until 1634, when T. Johnson produced a translation of his complete works; there were a number of subsequent editions of the works, but no separate issue of the midwifery part. But in 1612, a little book written in French in 1609 by Paré's pupil Jacques Guillemeau, was translated into English as *Child-birth, or the happy deliverie of women*. In this book the first description of podalic version, popularised by Paré in cases of emergency, appeared in English.[7]

Shortly after Paré's complete works were translated another much earlier work was published in English in 1637, namely Jacob Rueff's *The expert midwife*, which had appeared in Latin under the title of *De conceptu et generatione hominis* in 1554. This interesting little book had illustrations, including anatomical diagrams, which were rather oddly left unlabelled, because 'we accounted it a superfluous thing, to marke and point out every severall thing with Letters and Characters, because they are extant, and to be seene every where in the books of those which have written of Anatomies'.[8] It is particularly important for the depiction of embryonic development as it was envisaged at the time.

The next midwifery title to appear in the shops was that by Nicholas Culpeper, an apothecary who practised in Spitalfields, a writer of many popular medical books, and a determined opponent of Popery and the Royal College of Physicians, which he thought were tarred with the same monopolistic brush. His *Directory for midwives* was published in 1651. It contains nothing whatsoever about practical midwifery because, as Culpeper ingenuously admitted, he knew nothing about it; 'I have not medled with your Callings nor Manual Operations, lest I should discover my Ignorance like *Phormio* the Phylosopher, who having never seen Battel, undertook to read a Military Lecture before *Hanibal*.'[9] A later author described his book as 'desperately deficient . . . except he writ it for necessity, he could certainly have never been so sinful to have exposed it to the light'.[10] Culpeper also bore the full brunt of the objections to such books on grounds of decency, which were continually raised from *The birth of mankind* onwards. One of his critics told a story of 'a Gentleman and Scholars censure upon your Book, who perusing some passages in it in a booksellers shop, asked whether *Culpeper* made that obsceane book or no, and being answered he did, replied, truly *Culpeper* hath made Culpaper, paper fit to wipe ones breech withal'.[11]

William Harvey's work on obstetrics *De partu* was published in Latin in 1651 and in English in 1653. It appeared as part of his work on embryology, entitled *Anatomical exercitations, concerning the generation of living creatures. To which are added particular discourses of births, and of conceptions etc.* This work shows that Harvey, though not primarily an obstetrician, had practical knowledge of midwifery, and emphasises the value of Paré's work on the management of difficult labours.

In 1656 an anonymous work signed C. T. appeared; this was followed closely in 1659 by an almost identical work signed C. R. Both were entitled *The compleat midwife's practice enlarged* and contained material plagiarised from *Observations sur la stérilité*, written by the French Court midwife Louise Bourgeois. *Dr. Chamberlain's midwives practice* 1668, despite its preface signed P. C. was almost certainly not by Peter Chamberlen, but more likely by someone cashing in on the family reputation. If it had been by him it is hard to believe no reference would have been made to the family secret, the forceps. Certainly Hugh Chamberlen seized every opportunity to advertise them in the two versions he made of Mauriceau's work.

1671 saw the publication of no fewer than three new books for midwives. *The midwives book* was by Mrs Jane Sharp, who claimed to be a midwife of thirty years' standing, although if this is true it tends to show how ignorant midwives still were, and especially of Paré's important ideas. A similar ignorance is shown by James Wolveridge in *Speculum matricis*. This book adopts the form of an instructional dialogue between a doctor and a midwife, though the author was most likely unaware that the dialogue form, but between a midwife and her deputy, had previously been used by Edward Poeton in his earlier seventeenth-century book *The midwives deputie*.[12] The dialogue form for didactic works is of course a very old device indeed; *The midwives deputie* was probably never published however. William Sermon's book *The ladies companion, or the English midwife*, the third of the 1671 trio, is no more informative, and seems chiefly designed to advertise the author's famous cathartic and diuretic pills, only to be had of a certain bookseller.

Hugh Chamberlen's two versions of Mauriceau, *The accomplisht midwife* 1673, and *The diseases of women with child, and in child-bed* 1683 do not differ greatly from each other, though the second has a few additions. François Mauriceau was by far the most influential man-midwife of the day, and these are really the first satisfactory textbooks in English, since Percivall Willughby's book, *Observations in midwifery*, which was probably written in about 1672, was not published until the nineteenth century. It certainly postdates the three 1671 books, from which he quotes, and probably antedates the Mauriceau translations, which he does not mention. It is unfortunate that this book went unpublished, as it was firmly based on practical experience, anticipating the popular case-history style of many eighteenth-century writers. But three manuscript versions existed, so it may have been circulated among a small number of practitioners.

The anonymous *The English midwife enlarged* 1682, is clearly a publisher's pot-boiler, and is an amalgam of Wolveridge and Mauriceau, some passages copied verbatim. James McMath's *The expert midwife* 1694, was published in Edinburgh, presumably for a Scottish public, and is remarkable chiefly for its turgid style.

The two books published by John Pechey, *A general treatise of the diseases of maids, big-bellied women, child-bed women, and widows* 1696, and *The compleat midwife's practice enlarged* 1698, are heavily indebted to the previous anonymous works of 1656 and 1659, including the section copied from Louise Bourgeois, but with the addition of a new section purporting to be taken from the private papers of Sir Theodore de Mayerne, personal physician to Charles I. Pechey claimed to be a near relation of Sir Theodore. He was a member of the Royal College of Physicians, but was prosecuted by them for advertising cut-price attendance and medicine on a guaranteed 'no cure, no fee' basis, and also for not paying the college's fees. It is not known whether he practised as a man-midwife.

However Robert Barret's *A companion for midwives, childbearing women, and nurses* 1699, probably is by a man-midwife, since some case-material is introduced by way of example.

During the seventeenth century several other books appeared, intended less for midwives than for women in general, namely J. Sadler, *The sicke womans private looking-glass* 1636; N. Fontanus, *The womans doctour* 1652; the anonymous *A rich closet of physical secrets* probably also 1652;[13] N. Sudell, *Mulierum amicus, or the woman's friend* 1666; and R. Turner, *De morbis foemineis* 1686.

Throughout the sixteenth and seventeenth centuries there were also, written in English or translated into it, a large number of popular and semi-popular books on physic and surgery, often with sections relating to gynaecology and obstetrics, and often claiming to be expressly intended for midwives and surgeons as well as the general reader. There was a fair amount of opposition to be overcome to publishing such subjects in English, especially in the case of physic, since anyone with a claim to a good education could at this time read Latin.[14]

By the end of the seventeenth century however, the battle was largely over, since there was no law of copyright and thus nothing to prevent booksellers with an eye on a good popular market from publishing translations of anything they chose. Thus in 1682 T. Gibson wrote *The anatomy of humane bodies epitomiz'd* in English, 'to avoid the injury of a paltry Translator, if it should be well accepted. For we see there is no Man that publishes any thing in the Latin tongue, that is received with any applause, but presently some progging Book-seller or other finds out an indigent Hackney scribler to render it into English. But with what dis-reputation and abuse to the worthy Authors, every learned person cannot but observe'.

The principal books on midwifery in the early-eighteenth century were also translations, chiefly from French, where the surgeons were foremost in obstetrics until about the middle of the century, when English men-midwives began to be equally esteemed. Paul Portal's *La practique des accouchemens* 1685, was translated into English, in 1705, as *The compleat practice of men and women midwives.*[15] Hendrik van Deventer's Latin book of 1701 appeared in English in 1716 as *The art of midwifery improv'd*, and Pierre Dionis' French treatise in 1719 as *A general treatise of midwifery*. In 1746 M. Mauquest de la Motte's case-book was translated by Thomas Tomkyns, surgeon, as *A general treatise of midwifery*, originally published in French in 1722.

Three authors contributed about this time in English; John Maubray's *The female physician*, heavily indebted to Deventer, appeared in 1724, and Edmund Chapman's *A treatise on the improvement of midwifery; chiefly with regard to the operation* in 1733. The operation in question was the application of the obstetric forceps, first explained in this book. In 1734 the first illustration of the new instrument was made public in William Giffard's *Cases in midwifery*, published posthumously the year after Giffard's death. These latest books were more specifically designed for the male rather than the female midwife; a sign of the times and a foretaste of the future.

*Chapter Two*

# The Legacy of the Ancients, and William Harvey

At the beginning of the sixteenth century medical science was firmly based on the classical tradition of humoral medicine, especially on the works of Galen and the Hippocratic writings. Many of these texts had come down through the middle ages in Latin translations, and had been supplemented by material of Arabic origin, also in Latin translations.

The original Greek texts had recently been rediscovered, and there were high hopes that medicine would now free itself of all the errors which had crept in over the centuries and enshrine once more the pure teaching of Galen and Hippocrates. Medical thought was regarded as finished; humoral medicine, although it had no basis in reality, was such an internally logical construct that it offered explanations and cures for all diseases, and reasons for any question about anatomy and physiology.[1] Although large numbers of people unfortunately did die of their diseases, this was not seen as any sort of grounds for impugning the theory.

It is difficult now to conceive of the reverence accorded to the ancients and their writings. Anyone who advanced ideas contrary to their teaching was regarded as a dangerous iconoclast; but as the number of these heretics grew during the sixteenth and seventeenth centuries the structure gradually fell into disarray, beginning with anatomy, as a result of the important discoveries of the period, though humoral medicine lingered on as therapy well into the nineteenth century. It has been suggested that the social needs of doctor and patient were subserved by humoral medicine, and that it persisted because it rationalised and legitimated the physician's role.[2] Perhaps more importantly it provided a 'rational' basis for the then universal assumption of male superiority. Further, the new scientific facts which revealed the errors of the ancients in anatomy and physiology did not offer any alternative therapy, and neither doctor nor patient was likely to accept a position in which nothing could be cured.

The tenets of humoral medicine have often been described, but those aspects which are found in the obstetrical literature of our period must be described briefly here in order to demonstrate the nature and extent of the changes which came about at this time.

Broadly speaking, humoral medicine was based on the belief that everything was made up of four elements — earth, air, fire and water. These elements possessed qualities of cold, heat, dryness and moisture in different combinations and degrees. In the body there were four humours, also possessing these qualities, each being associated with a colour — blood with red, bile or choler with yellow, black bile or melancholy with black, and phlegm with white. These colours and properties largely formed the basis for diagnosis.

Every individual was born with his own particular complexion or constitution, in which one of the humours usually predominated over the others, and determined whether his temperament would be sanguine, choleric, melancholy or phlegmatic. As long as the individual's personal balance of humours was maintained the body was healthy, but when some influence altered the balance disease resulted. Cure consisted in deciding which way the humours were disordered, and redressing the balance on the principle of opposites. Thus a disease arising from phlegm, which is cold and moist, required purging and bleeding to take away the excess humour, and a regimen of hot dry foods and medicines to counteract it.

Although other causes of disease such as miasmata, adverse planetary influences and 'contagion' were recognised, even they produced their effects largely by acting upon the humours. Thus excessive menses might be caused by the blood being mixed with superfluous phlegm, melancholy or choler; or the expulsive faculty might be too strong and the retentive too weak, or the blood might be hot and sharp and corrode the vessels.[3]

Diagnosis of the peccant humour could be made in such diseases by dipping a cloth in the blood or discharge and noting the colour, 'which if it be red, it proceeds from bloud; if white, from *phlegme*, if yellow, it takes beginning from *choler*'.[4] In other cases the urine would be used to diagnose the peccant humour, though uroscopy was now much out of fashion with the learned.

Because diseases were not seen as separate clinical entities one disease could change into another depending on where the humours went and how they behaved. Suppression of the lochia in childbed, for example, might cause 'great difficulty of Breathing, stoppage at Stomach, palpitation of the Heart, *Syncopes*, Convulsions and

*Delirium*, and these Symptoms frequently prove Mortal to her. If the Suppression continues, there is a great danger of an Abscess in the Womb, or perhaps of a *Cancer* or Aposthumes in the lower Belly, Sciatica's, Lameness, or Inflammations, and Abscess of the Breasts, according as the Humours take there [sic] courses'.[5]

Treatment, if erroneous, could thus turn a disease into something worse by driving the humours on to some more vulnerable part, or by exasperating their bad qualities. The importance of the physician being properly schooled in the theory of humoral medicine was quite evident. So Willis observed that milk fever would go off by sweat and the lochia unless an error of management interfered, such as driving back the milk by topical applications, in which case worse symptoms would develop and it would turn into the much more dangerous puerperal fever.[6]

A course of physic was expensive, unpleasant, complicated and almost a full-time occupation for both patient and doctor. The patient kept his chamber and drank posset while the doctor prescribed remedies, beginning with the mild ones, and then if noticeable results were not very quickly produced going on to more drastic ones. The disease was attacked on all possible fronts by purging, clysters (enemas), vomits, bleeding, issues,[7] leeches, sweating, cupping, blistering, bathing, fomenting, fumigating and poulticing, by diet and by medicines of astonishing complexity, not only in ingredients, but in mode of presentation.

Bleeding was used both to evacuate the humour from the affected part, and to turn back its course in some more desirable direction. In uterine haemorrhage therefore 'let blood in the Arm in the first place . . . for unless you draw back the blood you can never stop it; as you must pump out the Water of a Ship before you can stop the leak'.[8]

Bleeding was so widely and generally used that perhaps a seventeenth century author may be allowed to explain the theory. When in a childbed patient chest symptoms arise 'we must mark whether the Fluxion [of humours] be only beginning . . . and very little blood be collected in the part. For then the inferior Veins are to be opened, that revulsion may be made to such opposite parts as are at greatest distance from the part affected, and by that means that preposterous motion of Humors may be stopped. But if the fluxion be already in good measure begun . . . the superior Veins are presently to be opened right against the Part affected, because such an Evacuation draws Blood out of the Part Affected . . . Neither need we fear, lest by taking blood from the upper Veins, we should draw the Course thereof from the womb [i.e.

stop the lochia] because in such Cases the superior parts of the Body do abound with blood. And although much blood be taken away, yet are not the Veins so emptied, that they should be forced to draw new blood from other parts'.[9]

Such reasoning totally fails to grasp that Harvey's observations on the circulation of the blood necessarily imply that blood cannot be taken from any one part in isolation, nor drawn to it. Indeed Harvey himself did not press his discovery so far, and bleeding continued long afterwards, partly because both doctor and patient needed *some* action to be taken, and partly because both were persuaded that cures actually were frequently effected thereby. As Guillemeau confidently stated, in cases of uterine haemorrhage 'the most singular, and presentest remedie is to let bloud in the arme, which I haue seen tried by the most learned Physitions of our age, with very good successe: For there is no meanes, that makes better revulsion, and drawes the bloud sooner from the place, to which it floweth, then opening of a veine'.[10]

The humours were thought to be fluids that moved about the body along with the blood, which ebbed and flowed in response to various faculties, of which there were many — expulsive, retentive, attractive and so on. It was chiefly in terms of these faculties that physiological activity was described. Thus the stomach attracted food by the attractive faculty, retained it by the retentive while the first concoction took place, and then expelled the residue by the expulsive.

Concoction, as digestion was called, was envisaged as a three-stage process; an actual cooking of the food by the natural heat of the liver warming the stomach like a pot. Natural heat was that which chiefly distinguished the living from the dead, death being a loss of all natural heat, and therefore a cessation of all vital processes.

In the fifteenth century concoction was described in this way: 'all the meat & dry*n*k that is recevid goethe into the stomak & ther it is sodden and defied & all that is great & not profitable passethe downe to the bowell called longauo*n* and that y[t] bidethe in the stomake turnythe into mylk and so passethe into the lyv*er* and ther abidethe till he be defied sodden & well clensed & all that is not p*ro*fitable passethe to the reynes & into the bledd*re* & so owt & that is called uryne symple but that is good that abydethe in the lyver & ther turnethe to bloud & so fro*m* thens It passethe to all the humours of the bodye and nouryshethe the lyff'.[11]

In the seventeenth century the concoctions were still described in much the same terms.[12] According to Culpeper the third concoction turned blood into flesh, evidently by depositing nutriment in the various parts it came to. In women, the excrement of the third concoction gathered about the uterus and was purged out each month as the menses. Sweat and 'fuliginous vapours' were also the waste products of the third concoction and were excreted through the pores of the skin. There were also other mysterious breathing holes and secret passages through which vapours and wind could pass, as well as by the veins. In the brain a further concoction turned vital spirit into animal spirit, while in the testicles blood was concocted into generative seed, and in the breasts into milk.

Although William Harvey's great discovery of the circulation of the blood was published in 1628, it was a further half century before any use of it or even reference to it appeared in an English midwifery book. Older views still prevailed in the more popular writers; according to Wolveridge veins originated from the liver, whereas arteries arose from the heart.[13] Sharp agreed: 'It will be needful that you should know that the fountain of *blood* is the *Liver* . . . and the Liver by the Veins disperse the blood through the Body'.[14]

The blood could be thickened and obstructed and cause diseases; thus the maids' disease, chlorosis, was caused by 'obstructions of the Veins, of the Liver, Spleen, Mesentery, and especially the womb, whereby the whole passage of blood is hindred . . . and . . . turns to the upper parts and oppresseth the Heart, Liver, Spleen, Midriff and other parts; destroying natural heat, and bringing evil concoction in the bowels'.[15]

Suppression of the menses caused disease because 'the suppressed bloud wanders up and down the veins, & begets obstructions, changing the colour of the body, and causing feavers'.[16] Furthermore, the right testicle produced hotter seed than the left because 'it receives more pure and Vital blood from the hollow Vein and the great Artery then the left doth, which receives onely a watry bloud from the Emulgent Vein'.[17] In Rueff the arteries are *called* veins: 'For as *Vena cava* is the originall, fountain and spring of all the veines by which the body attracteth and draweth to it the whole nutriment of blood: Even so, from this great veine, *Aorta*, are derived all the pulsive, moving, and beating-veines, on every side dispersing & pouring forth vital spirit thorowout the whole body'.[18]

But in Mauriceau's work the newer view appeared: 'the Arteries convey the Blood, for as much as the circular Motion, which is made continually in all living Animals, shows us, that they alone are capable of doing it, and not the Veins, which serve only to reconduct to the Heart, the Blood which is not evacuated'.[19] Working on this information he correctly ascribed the cause of varicose veins in pregnancy to obstruction of the return flow to the heart by the weight of the uterus, where earlier authors had been obliged to regard it as a weakness of the expulsive faculty; it followed that medical treatment was less likely to succeed than rest and supporting bandages.[20] Pechey, in 1698, similarly rejected the old idea that the arteries and veins going to the testicles mixed the blood together and concocted it into seed: 'since the knowledge of the Circulation of the Blood, this Opinion has been rejected; for the blood in the Arteries goes down towards the Stones, and that in the veins ascends from them'.[21]

Yet these same authors, who clearly understood these implications of the circulation of the blood, could not take the further step of realising that the rationale of blood-letting was thereby undermined. Mauriceau himself advised bleeding in the arm for uterine haemorrhage, and thought that if pain in the breasts during pregnancy was due to excess blood flowing to them it was much better to evacuate it by bleeding in the arm, than to turn or drive it back on some other part of the body.

According to the ancients the function of respiration was to cool the heart, the lungs acting simply as bellows. Riverius stated that women in hysterical fits did not breathe because the heart was already so cooled by venemous vapours that there was no need of respiration. That there was a link between respiration and the blood was dimly understood, though nobody yet, including Harvey, knew about the function of blood-borne oxygen in sustaining life.[22] Harvey had however observed that although a newborn baby needs air immediately it could not be for refrigeration, for 'the *Heat* within him . . . is rather inflamed, then quenched by the Aire'.[23]

The practical implications of this observation were clear to the better surgeons, and reinforced by experience. Read noted that if the umbilical cord prolapsed during the birth, the baby was in great danger of death unless promptly delivered, 'because the Blood can be no longer vivified and renewed by circulation, as it has continual need'. The coming first of the afterbirth must similarly be a grave emergency for the child, 'standing then in need of breathing by the Mouth, the Blood being no longer vivified by the preparation made in the Burthen, the use and function of which then ceases, from the instant it is separated from the vessels of the Womb, to which it was joyned'.[24] Until the ancients' physiology had been thus far corrected the remedy for the stillbirth of many babies in such circumstances — immediate operative delivery — could hardly be found.

*Chapter Three*

# The Legacy of the Ancients, and the Anatomists

The fifteenth and sixteenth century rediscovery of Galen's works, in particular the *Anatomical procedures*, which had previously been known only in textually-corrupt later versions,[1] along with other influences, stimulated interest in anatomy as the basis for medical studies, and soon a new approach to the study and teaching of the subject was adopted, especially in Italy. Oxford and Cambridge unfortunately remained trammelled by mediaeval approaches, and produced no anatomist of note. Harvey, whose work has already been mentioned, owed much to his studies at Padua in the days after Vesalius's reforms.

Vesalius as a young man was appalled by the teaching of anatomy at Padua: 'everything is wrongly taught in the schools, and days are wasted in ridiculous questions so that in such confusion less is presented to the spectators than a butcher in his stall could teach a physician'.[2] Herein it differed little from the teaching at other universities of the period, where medical students spent their time reading Latin translations of parts of Galen, Hippocrates and the *Canon* of Avicenna, and scoring points in formal 'school' disputations. There was no clinical teaching whatever, anatomies were not frequent and were somewhat perfunctory affairs where the body was opened by a menial assistant and the lecturer described the parts, not from the body, but from one of the approved texts. Even Mondino de' Luzzi, who in the early-fourteenth century broke with custom so far as to dissect personally, failed to correct some egregious errors in Galen, because his purpose was demonstration, not research.

An unhealthy veneration for authority was characteristic of late mediaeval thought, in medicine as in other branches of philosophy. Indeed, although the new experimental anatomy of the sixteenth century soon proved that the ancients, and Galen in particular, had made notable errors, there were still a few diehards who could not shake off this attitude at the end of the seventeenth century. One author, in 1684, tells the story of a public anatomy lecturer and devoted disciple of Aristotle, who when shown the vena cava arising from the liver (although Aristotle said all veins arose from the heart) refused to believe his eyes, 'because, said he, it is much more easy for our Senses to be sometimes deceived, than for the Great and Soveraign *Aristotle* ever to have faln into any Error'.[3]

Much more characteristic of the spirit of the seventeenth century however was Culpeper's comment, 'my opinion is, that he is not very wise that altogether neglects Authors, but he is a fool in grain that beleeves them before his own eyes.'[4] Harvey, although he thought it unbecoming to slight the ancients, also thought right-minded men do not 'think it base to change their opinion, if truth and open demonstration do perswade them, and [do] not think it shameful to desert their errors, though they be never so antient'.[5]

Discoveries in physiology, because they were more dependent on reasoning and less on visible evidence, tended to arouse differences of opinion, and to take a long time to gain general acceptance, but even here the methods of the anatomists were a model to imitate wherever possible. It was this kind of proof that Harvey sought in his own work: 'I have not endeavoured from causes and probable principles to demonstrate my propositions, but as of higher authority, to establish them by appeals to sense and experiment after the manner of the anatomists'.[6]

Much work has been done tracking down the authors of the very numerous discoveries in anatomy and physiology of the period, but in the following pages I shall concentrate on those ideas which found their way into the vernacular textbooks intended for practitioners, including midwives, and may thus be supposed to have influenced actual practice and popular thought.

Although the number of books in English on anatomy, or aspects of it, suggests that there was much interest in it at quite a popular level, opportunities for anatomical discovery, and even basic instruction, were particularly limited in England. Midwives and the public generally had few or no opportunities to learn anatomy at first hand, although there were travelling exhibitions of anatomical specimens to be seen.[7]

Even the medical profession was hampered in this country by popular prejudice against dissection. Willughby noted that 'In France, and the Low Countries, they have many privileges, and customes which we cannot obtain in England. They open dead bodies, without any mutterings of their friends. Should one of us desire such a thing, an odium of inhumane cruelty would bee upon us by the vulgar, and common people'.[8] In France it was indeed mandatory for women dying in labour to be opened, with the object of baptizing the child if it should be alive.[9]

Nevertheless individuals in England did succeed in obtaining specimens, performing post mortem examinations, and sometimes in demonstrating their findings. Harvey performed a post mortem on a particular friend of his, and kept as specimens some foetal bones ejected from an abscess, and a small embryo, which was eviscerated and kept for some months in cold water. Sharp claimed to have seen an ovary on one occasion, and Culpeper to have seen the anatomy of a woman who died undelivered, but both clearly regarded these as exceptional opportunities.[10]

Medical men seem to have had more opportunities than Willughby's comment suggests in some cases. Glisson made reference to frequent autopsies which he had made on rachitic bodies, and based his clinical deductions about the disease on these.[11] Several communications to the Royal Society in its early days concern such investigations. In William Giffard's practice a highly abnormal case occurred in which a foetus developed in a sacculus and was born per anum. Giffard, along with Mr Nourse, surgeon to St Bartholomew's hospital, dissected the mother, and the report together with the organs was presented to the Royal Society. The President, Sir Hans Sloane, had drawings made of the parts which are reproduced in Giffard's book.[12]

Nevertheless the progress of obstetrics might have been hastened if the dissection of women dying in pregnancy and labour had been more frequently practised. It is certainly true that the female reproductive organs were less well described than either the male reproductive organs or those other organs which are common to both sexes and where observations made in the male subject were equally valid for the female. This followed from the relative unavailability of female cadavers.

*Chapter Four*

# The Female Reproductive System

According to humoral theory the chief difference between the sexes was in the degree of natural heat they possessed. Men were far hotter than women. Heat was the cause of vigour, strength, courage and intellect, and thus it followed that men were naturally superior to women in all these respects; 'so that a woman is so much less perfect then a man, by how much her heat is lesser and weaker than his'.[1] Women's seed was watery and cold, men's was finer and more spirituous and therefore more highly endowed with active procreative principle.[2] Women had more blood in their bodies than men, but it was of a much inferior quality.[3] It was therefore a scientific fact that 'a Female is a thing more imperfect then a Male'.[4]

Anatomically, however, the ancients held that there was virtually no difference between the sexes, the man's penis and testicles being exactly analogous to the uterus and ovaries, but situated outside the body because of men's greater heat. According to Paré the generative parts of men and women differ 'onely in situation and use. For that which man hath apparent without, that women have hid within'.[5] This situation of the organs was partly to keep men more chaste, because birds and such male creatures as had their testicles inside the body were well known to be more salacious. Likewise men with undescended testicles were notoriously 'most excessive prone to lechery'.

As the anatomical description of the parts became increasingly detailed however, differences of opinion arose about which male part corresponded to which female, and by the late seventeenth century this idea was on the way out. The anatomist Bartholin, whose anatomy was translated into English in 1668, expressly denied it.[6] Although she accepted the idea that the female parts were like the male reversed, Mrs Sharp did not think the similarity was so great as to enable a sex change to take place, and Dr Chamberlain also denied any such change had ever happened, as it was rumoured to have.

Women of a naturally hot manly temperament, who did not

menstruate, were much healthier than moister women and really needed no treatment, except that they would then be sterile. Therefore 'Such as are robust and of a manly Constitution must by all means be reduced to a womanly state; that they may become fit for generation, they must forbear strong Meats and Labour, and the Courses must be forced, and by Bleeding and Purging and the like, the habit of the Body must be rendred cold and moist'.[7]

The uterine parts had been fairly well described by Soranus and other ancient authors, but later the idea arose that the uterus was divided into seven cells: there were three on the right for males, three on the left for females, and in the middle one either the seed was not retained or a hermaphrodite was engendered. The seven-celled uterus, although the less erudite authors took it to be a Galenic error, perhaps originated in the thirteenth-century *Liber physiognomiae* of Michael Scot, which was printed in 1477.[8] Mondino de' Luzzi repeated the idea and it appears in some of the fifteenth-century English *Libri Trotuli*, though not in the original *Trotula*.

Da Carpi had refuted this idea early in the sixteenth century, and published drawings of the uterus showing it clearly as one-celled. Galen had in fact described the uterus as double, but whether he was referring to the bi-cornuate uterus found in some animals, or to the human uterus including the Fallopian tubes, is by no means clear.[9]

None of the midwifery books still taught that the uterus was seven-celled, indeed the 1545 *Birth of mankind* expressly denied it;[10] nevertheless Culpeper and Sharp both said many contemporary midwives did believe this. Some sort of duality was ascribed to the uterus long after the seven cells had become a notorious error, but whether this was due to following Galen, or influenced unduly by the Hippocratic idea that males lay on the right and females on the left, is uncertain. The belief that the uterus was analogous to the scrotum, and the vagina to the penis, may also have influenced the representation of these parts, as the illustrations in Paré, after Vesalius, demonstrate.

Paré said the womb was divided into two recesses, but not physically separate. Sharp said 'It hath but one hollow Cell, yet this at the bottom is in some manner divided into two, as if there were two wombs fastened to one neck', so that 'Perhaps it is no error to say the Wombs are two, because there are two cavities like two hollow hands touching one the other, both covered with one Pannicle, and both ending in one channel'.[11] Her book was not illustrated, and this description is not altogether clear, but most likely no more was intended than is shown by the section through the uterus in Paré, where there is a little dividing wall at the fundus.

The ancients thought of the womb as an animal eager for young and turning spiteful if frustrated, an idea said to originate in Plato's dialogue *Timaeus*. It was believed to open and suck in male seed in conception, to have voluntary motion, and to be much affected by smells. All these ideas were still current in the seventeenth century, and the two latter in the eighteenth, although a somewhat more sophisticated interpretation was put on them. Guillemeau explained that 'the Matrice hath voluntary motion, towards euery part . . . But these situations, and changings of place must not be vnderstood, in an exact sence. For it is vnlikely, nay impossible, that the Matrice, should so run from one side of the body to another, that it should altogether leaue his owne place'.[12]

The idea that the uterus was affected by smells also gradually became less naïvely understood. Dr Chamberlain pointed out that it could not actually *smell* anything, but was nevertheless affected by a subtle vapour arising from strong-smelling things.[13] As late as 1755, *Aristotle's experienced midwife* restated the 'certain Truth, that the Womb flies from all stinking, and to all sweet things'. These notions were influential in diagnosis and therapy. Also influencing therapy was the idea that the uterus was the chief route by which women eliminated bad humours, and was thus 'the common *Sink* of the Body'.

The female organs had not so far been represented in side view, and it was late in the seventeenth century before it was realised clearly that the uterus and vagina do not continue in a straight line, but that the uterus and cervix are tilted at an angle. This was important in practice however, and midwives' ignorance of this led to their attempts at digital examination sometimes proving uninformative. Sharp was following the old view when she described the fundus, cervix and vagina as lying directly in line with each other, 'for the Seed goeth in a streight line from the neck to the bottom'.[14]

The cervix was believed to be sensitive to stimuli, it also 'opens naturally in Copulation, in voiding menstruous blood and in childbirth; but at other times, especially when a woman is with Child, it shuts so close, that the smallest needle cannot get in but by force'.[15] The opening of the cervix was believed to be part of the orgasmic experience for women, because it only happened if the womb was sufficiently heated and receptive. Therefore frigidity was a cause of sterility, for if the cervix did not open, clearly it could not receive the seed. Fortunately however 'in some Women the wombe is so greedy, and lickerish that it doth euen come down to meet nature, sucking, and (as it were) snatching the same, though it remaine only about the mouth and entrance of the outward orifice thereof'.[16] This, since no one had yet seen spermatozoa, explained how conception could occur even in frigid women, and in those with physical impediments to the entry of the male organ.

The vagina was known to be wrinkled, which enabled it to suit any man; Sharp somewhat tartly observed it 'is fit for any Yard: yet I have heard a *French* man complain sadly, that when he first married his Wife, it was no bigger nor wider than would fit his turn, but now it was grown as a Sack; Perhaps the fault was not the womans but his own, his weapon shrunk and was grown too little for the scabbard'.[17]

Because it was generally agreed that women had seed, which they must emit in orgasm for conception, the clitoris was assigned an important role in generation, and it was believed without it a woman would not only have no desire for copulation or pleasure in it, but she would not conceive by it either. Despite the ovum theory which had by then gained general acceptance, at the popular level *Aristotle's masterpiece* was repeating the same thing in 1755.

The muscular nature of the uterine wall was also important for conception, because it closed in on the seed to retain it while the two seeds mixed together. It had three sorts of fibres, some to attract the seed, some to retain it, and some for expulsion if necessary. This apparently fairly clear idea of the uterine muscles is not really so, but follows Galen's idea that not only the uterus but many other organs had these fibres, and that they accounted for the movement of blood in the veins and food in the alimentary canal.[18] The role of the uterine muscles in labour was not fully realised until the eighteenth century, as earlier authors believed the foetus played the more important part.

There was a long-standing difference of opinion as to whether the wall of the uterus grew thicker or thinner as pregnancy progressed, a point of practical importance affecting the depth of the incision in the performance of post mortem caesarean section to save the child. Chamberlain, Sharp and Pechey all said it got thicker the more it was extended, Deventer that it stayed the same and Mauriceau, Read and Dionis believed that it got thinner. Mauriceau declared 'it is not above . . . the thickness of half a Crown, although they have all sang to us, that by divine Providence and a Miracle, the more 'tis extended with the Child, the thicker it grows, which is absolutely false; it being only true, that it is at that time a little thicker at the place where the Burthen cleaves'.[19] Chapman noted that at one autopsy he found the womb very thin compared to others he had seen, and thought that was probably the reason for the lack of agreement, 'every one speaking as he himself has happened to find it'.[20]

Mauriceau was clear that it was the contraction of the uterus that controlled haemorrhage from the placental site, an important point in the management of ante-partum haemorrhage.[21]

The fundus of the uterus was thought to contain 'cotyledons', which were the mouths of blood-vessels through which menstrual blood passed, as well as blood for nourishing the foetus.[22] Vesalius doubted this, and in the 1555 *Fabrica* demonstrated that true cotyledons are found only in ruminants.[23] Mauriceau clearly stated that they are found only in horned beasts, but in 1699 Barret stuck to the older idea: 'In Women not with Child, the Menstrual Blood always flows through the Arteries . . . In the time of flowing they are opened and gape. They resemble Cups or Saucers, call'd, *Acetabula* or *Cotyledones*. To these, when a Woman is with Child, the *Placenta* is join'd'.[24]

Harvey noted that the uterine wall changed in texture in preparation for conception, and Bartholin and Dionis that it was thicker at menstruation; 'for the Blood brought thither in abundance at that time entring its Substance, swells it; but it grows thinner again, as these *Purgations* go off'.[25] This was the nearest to the modern explanation that anyone came during that time, but it did not replace the older view that the blood came from the arteries, as both Bartholin and Dionis stated elsewhere.

The idea that the male and female genitals were essentially the same necessarily implied that the ovaries contained and ejaculated seed. Indeed all through our period the same words, 'testicles' or 'stones', were used for both male and female gonads. And this despite increasing attention, following Harvey's work on generation, to the idea that the female testicles did not contain seed, but were a cluster of eggs. Until the late seventeenth century however, by far the most widely-accepted view was that they did contain seed, which was emitted during orgasm and mixed with the male seed on conception.

This idea, coupled with the belief that menstrual blood came from the arteries at the fundus, led to all sorts of speculation about the vessels through which seed and menstrual blood passed, especially during pregnancy when the womb was closed. It was evident that since they could not come through the womb without causing abortion, there must be some sort of by-pass. These imaginary vessels are marked 'kk' on the uterus illustration in Paré. Although Dionis pointed out in 1724 that these vessels cannot be found in human bodies, *Aristotle's experienced midwife* in 1755 still insisted there were vessels at the cervix which let out excess blood and humours during pregnancy, so that the cervix need not open.

The vessels by which non-pregnant women menstruated and ejaculated seed were also, not surprisingly, far from easy to identify. Thus the round and ovarian ligaments were taken to be ejaculatory vessels by some, while the Fallopian tubes were said to be merely ligaments by others. Rueff evidently thought they were ligaments: 'Further in the same part, on the right and left side, two hornes, as it were, do bosse out . . . To those Ligaments, or stay-bands, the testicles or stones are annexed and combined'.[26] Riverius also thought there was no passage through 'that blind Vessel, which from *Fallopius* the finder or first Observer thereof is called *Fallopious* his Trumpet, becavse he likened the same to the broad end of a Trumpet'.[27] Indeed in making this comparison Fallopius himself was referring only to their shape, since he did not realise they were patent.[28] Our term 'Fallopian tube', though more accurately descriptive, is a happy mistranslation.

The question where menstrual blood came from puzzled Vesalius; 'how this occurs and through what veins in particular . . . perhaps you are in doubt like me'.[29] Pechey said the veins and arteries of the female genitals were very large, partly 'Because that the monthly purgations are poured through those veins; for the flowers must not come only out of the Womb, but out of the neck of the Womb also. Whence it happens, that Women with Child do sometimes continue their purgations, because that though the womb be shut up, yet the passages in the neck of the womb are open'.[30] Dr Chamberlain also thought that although the cervix normally opened during coitus, in pregnancy it did not open, but the female seed was voided instead by other passages leading to the vagina. However according to Pechey the ligaments of the womb 'which have bin accounted ejaculatory Vessels, either are not to be found at all, or are found unfit for such an Office' and it is the Fallopian tubes which conduct the ovum to the uterus.[31]

In contrast to the confusion surrounding the seed-carrying vessels, there was general agreement up to the mid-seventeenth century that the ovaries *were* female testicles, albeit 'much colder and lesser than Mens; which is the reason that they beget a thin and watry Seed'.[32] Vesalius and others had actually seen the Graafian follicles and the corpus luteum, but thought that they were pathological.[33] Dr Chamberlain said that women's testicles were not exactly the same as mens': 'their upper face is unequall, as if they were many small *glandules*'. In health they contained a wheyish humour, but when sick it was yellow and of a very evil scent, frequently causing fits of the mother.[34] According to Riverius, the anatomist Riolanus had seen the stones of hysterical virgins 'greater than his Fist, strouting with wheyish seed'.[35] Thus both the normal cyclic changes in the ovary and abnormal cystic conditions were taken by anatomists looking for female seed as evidence that there was such a thing.

Although the ovum theory was not long in gaining credence, Mauriceau to the end of his life refused to believe it, or that women had no seed; 'a great absurdity to believe: for the contrary may easily be discovered, by seeing the Spermatick Vessels and Testicles of a fruitful Woman, appointed for this use, which are wholly filled with this seed, which in coition they discharge as well as Men'.[36] But Pechey decided in favour of the new theory; women's stones, he said, contain 'several little bladders full of a clear Liquor . . . *Galen* and *Hypocrates*, and their followers, imagine the Liquor contained in these Bladders to be Seed; but from Dr. *Harvey* downwards, many learned Physicians, and Anatomists, have denied that Women have Seed . . . We must therefore agree with that new, but necessary Opinion, that supposes these little Bladders to contain nothing of Seed . . . they are truly Eggs, Analogous to those of Fowl, and other Creatures, and that the Stones so called are not truly so, nor have any such Office, as those of Men, but are indeed an *Ovarium* . . . from whence one or more, as they are fecundated by the Mans Seed, separate, and are convey'd into the womb by the *Fallopian tubes*'.[37]

This revolutionary idea was to have a profound effect in time on the way the female role in sexual intercourse and generation was viewed, and unhappily paved the way for the indifference to women's sexuality found in the nineteenth century.

*Chapter Five*

# Sexuality and Conception

Especially on the subjects of conception, sexuality, pregnancy and menstruation during this time, it is often impossible to tell whether a scientific 'fact' has passed into common knowledge and become a generally received opinion, or an existing popular belief or practice has been rationalised and authenticated by giving it a 'scientific' explanation.

But as a rule of thumb, however implausible an idea may seem now to us, if it was believed to have a rational and factual basis it was a scientific fact to contemporaries. If on the other hand it was denied, or doubted and said to be held by the common people, it was not. Thus it was a fact, as we shall see, that a child born at seven months could survive, but not at eight months, that peas and beans were good for impotence, and that the length of the penis depended on the length the navel-string was cut. It was only a common belief however that 'well hung Men are the greatest Blockheads'.[1] But there was certainly a large area of overlap between scientific fact and common knowledge, and a marked tendency for the scientific facts of one generation to become the old wives' tales of later generations.

A somewhat ambivalent attitude to sex prevailed in the seventeenth century, though the midwiferies contain a minimum of moralising. McMath said people copulate 'chiefly, from that signal *Delite*, and enchanting *Pleasure* found therein . . . For else how could man, so noble a *Creature*, make any attrectation of these *Obscoene parts*, which (for being so *Foulsome*, are turned down into the *Vilest Room*, in a manner the *Sink* of the *Body*) much less court, accept, or indulge to this *Embrace*, so filthy a *Fact* . . . What Woman also, would else impair her *Health* . . . in *Breeding*, *Bearing* and *bringing* up of *Children*, if not bewitched to this incredible pleasure excited in *Coition*'.[2]

Because for the greater part of this period it was believed that women had to emit seed in order to conceive, much attention was paid to the anatomy and physiology of sexual pleasure. Columbus and

Fallopius gave the first anatomical descriptions of the clitoris, but it would be naïve to imagine they actually discovered it, or that their statements that it was the chief seat of sexual pleasure in women came as a great revelation. Not only the clitoris however, but the carunculae myrtiformes, labia minora, vagina, cervix and Bartholin's glands were each, according to at least one author, designed chiefly for sexual excitement.

The clitoris was assigned a vital role in conception, and also credited with less legitimate uses: 'commonly it is but a small sprout, lying close hid under the Wings, and not easily felt, yet sometimes it grows so long that it hangs forth at the slit like a Yard, and will swell and stand stiff if it be provoked, and some lewd women have attempted to use it as men do theirs . . . but I never heard but of one in this Country'.[3] Bartholin referred to such women as 'Rubsters', and Dionis observed 'there are some lascivious Women, who by *Friction* of this Part, receive so great Pleasure, that they care not for Men'.[4] In mentioning such matters as masturbation and lesbianism authors in this period adopt a much more neutral tone than do Victorian authors, who tend to either censor such topics or treat them in a heated and hysterical manner. I take this as evidence that Stuart opinion was less censorious and guilt-ridden about such things.

Dr Chamberlain explained how the clitoris by attrition communicated lustful imaginations to the ligaments and thence to the leading vessels of the seed, and thus stimulated women to emit their seed. So strong was the belief in female seed that women, the same as men, could have nocturnal pollutions 'merely by the Force of *Imaginary* VENERY: Especially among *Salacious Women*, a *Seminal Fluxion* may happen upon many different occasions'.[5]

Thus the relative slowness to arousal of cold women, which meant the cervix did not open soon enough to receive the man's seed, nor were they stimulated to emit their own seed, was a possible cause of sterility. This might be due to physical causes such as an unnaturally cold disposition of the womb itself, or to emotional ones such as 'hatred between Man and Wife, whereby the Woman having an aversion for such pleasure does not supply Spirits sufficient to make the Genital parts turgent at the time of Copulation; nor does the Womb kindly meet the Seed, and draw it into its Cavity, from whence and from mixture of both the Seeds, Conception arises'.[6] Parents were advised not to marry off their children to partners against their inclination, on pain of having no descendants. Husbands were admonished about the importance of foreplay and caresses, and also not to withdraw too quickly lest the seed catch cold.

There was no sudden change of mind on this matter even after it was realised that the moisture perceived by the woman was not seed but came from 'two certain little holes or pits, wherein is contained a serous humour; which being pressed out in the act of copulation, does not a little add to the pleasure thereof. This is the humour with which women do moisten the top of a mans Yard; not the Seed, but a humour proper to the place, voided out by the Womb'.[7]

All the same, it began to be plain that women did not need to be sexually aroused in order to conceive. La Vauguion declared 'we see every day, that some are impregnated without emission of Seed, or receiving the least Pleasure', thus giving the lie to the common belief that women never conceived upon a rape. This view was held by some authors however, and persisted even into the nineteenth century.[8]

Nor did the ovum theory of conception suddenly affect the belief that women needed orgasm to conceive, despite the gradual realisation that it was not essential in the way it used to be thought. Dionis, although committed to the ovum theory, still regarded it as important for conception 'that both Sexes emit at the same time: for tho that which is call'd the Seed of the Woman serves only to give her more Pleasure, yet it shows that the Womb is heated', which makes it contract on the man's seed, thrusting it into the Fallopian tubes which then carry it to the ovaries.[9] 'Love-Frolicks and Sporting not only put the Seed into Motion, but . . . makes them frisk up and down in their Reservatories' he maintained.

Even at the end of this period, and long after the ovum theory was widely known and accepted, *Aristotle's experienced midwife*, evidently quoting a popular view, said 'Pleasure and Delight, say they, is double in Women, to what it is in Men: For as the Delight of Men in Copulation, consists chiefly in the Emission of the Seed, so Women are delighted both in the Emission of their own, and the Reception of the Man's'; although it no longer had a scientific foundation 'the good Women themselves . . . positively affirm they are sensible of the Emission of their Seed in those Engagements'.[10] It was also strongly believed that women whose sexual needs were not satisfied were in danger of illness.

The male was considered to be able for procreation unless his parts were physically defective, or he was impotent. Impotence was not thought to be a mental or emotional problem, but purely physical, although erection was believed to be partly caused by imagination. Usually however it was effected partly by muscles, partly by pressure of seed, and partly by wind. In these cases impotence might be helped by eating 'windy meats' such as peas and beans. The corpus spongiosum of the penis had been described by anatomists, and Paré stated that it was filled with gross and black blood, which when 'provoked with a venereall fire' swelled up and erected the member. By the time Dionis wrote he did not discount the role of muscles and spirits, but thought nevertheless that blood was the principal cause of erection.

Defect of the parts included the penis being the wrong size, 'because the men be halfe geldinges, & haue a very short yard, so that they can not cast their seede into the innermost place of the matrice';[11] worse still, some men, but chiefly fools, had members so long that they were useless for generation.[12] Either of these defects might have been the midwife's fault for cutting the navel-string the wrong length, 'by reason of the Ligament coming from the Navel to the bottom of the Bladder; which if it be too much abreviated, draws up the Bladder, and consequently shortens the Yard'.[13]

So long as the female seed concept survived, the man was also obliged to ensure the woman's satisfaction, as we have seen. Thus barrenness might occur 'when there is no impediment of either side; except onely in the manner of the act: as when in the emission of the seed, the man is quicke and the woman too slow, whereby there is not a concurse of both seeds at the same instant, as the rules of conception require'.[14]

Because the seed had to go in a straight line, it was darkly hinted that 'Apish waies and manners of Copulation, hinder Conception'. The most fertile time was just after the menstrual period, when the womb was cleansed and dry, or just before, when there was plenty of matter for the formation and nutrition of the embryo. However women, unlike animals, could copulate and conceive at any time.

Some writers suggested that the stock of mankind could be improved if parents would apply themselves in the sexual act to ensure the conception of male, not female, children; 'for the Female, through the cold and moist of their Sex, cannot be indowed with so profound a judgement: We find indeed that they talke with appearance of knowledge in sleight and easie matters, but seldom reach any farther than to a sleight superficial smattering in any deep Science'.[15] In order to achieve this desirable result parents should ensure that the seeds of both parties fell into the right side of the womb.

We have already seen that the right testicle was believed to receive hotter blood than the left: 'And this stone is said to beget Boyes: and the left is the more colder, because it receives a more impure, and serous blood from the emulgent vein, making this stone more apt for the procreation of the Female'.[16] Apparently this was a well known fact, although scientists were beginning to doubt it. The anatomist Bartholin said it was a 'common Saying, Wenches are begot by the left Stone in the left side of the Womb; Boys by the right Stone in the right side . . . But I am not of Opinion, that wenches are alwaies begotten by the left Stone, and that it receives a colder sort of Seed'.[17] Early in the seventeenth century Guillemeau advised tying off the left testicle if a son was wanted and the right if a daughter, as farmers did with livestock. Evidently this was still commonly believed at the end of the century; Mauriceau explained that it could not be true: 'if they know after what manner the blood is circulated, they would . . . know that the Seed of both Testicles is the same exactly, being made of the same blood, brought to them . . . by the two Arteries, which arise out of the trunck *Aorta* . . . therefore those Husbandmen abuse themselves, in knitting up one of the testicles of their Bulls according as they desire either Males or Females'.[18] Nevertheless in 1724 Maubray still thought it probable that if the seed fell into the right side of the womb, from the right testicle of the man, a boy would be conceived.

A robust insistence on mutual pleasure was maintained throughout this period despite a variety of opinions about conception. Of the two theories about conception most important in this period, the first was dominant up to the publication in 1651 of Harvey's book on generation. After this Harvey's ovum theory gradually gained ground, and by 1755 had pride of place in even the most popular literature, though without entirely effacing the old ideas.

The older theory held that conception arose from the material union of two substances, one from the male, one from the female. The newer theory held that only the female contributed materially to the conception, but that the male supplied an essential impetus, without which the female contribution remained inert. There were other theories, but one or other of these two, and sometimes both, was generally presented to the readers of the midwiferies as fact.[19]

Mentioned by some authors — only to be condemned — was an eccentric idea, the reverse of Harvey's, representing an ancient view that the female did not contribute materially to the conception, but merely provided a nidus and nutriment. The adherents of this notion were stigmatised as atheistical fools and idle coxcombs. According to Bartholin, Paracelsus and others less famous 'have contrariwise been perswaded that a Child may be generated out of the Mothers womb: but no body will be forward to believe them, unless they could shew us some example . . . For that a little child should be made in a Glass of a Mans Seed and Menstrual Blood, placed in Horse-dung, it hath never been my hap to see as yet, and it ought to be doubted, because the Experiment cannot be made'.[20]

The two main theories had different explanations for such questions as to how women with physical impediments to penetration could conceive; how sex was determined; how offspring take the likeness of their parents; and how multiple births occur.

According to the two seeds theory, the 'greedy womb' explained conception without actual penetration. However this was regarded as highly exceptional at least, and the usual view was that 'it is not sufficient that the Man's Yard enter the *Vagina*, which is the anti-chamber to the Womb: for, if in the act of copulation, he knocks at the door, which is the internal orifice, and it be not opened, all is to no purpose'.[21]

According to the two seeds theory once male and female seeds had entered the womb it closed, 'after which it reduceth by its heat, from power into action, the several faculties, which are in the seeds it contains, making use of the Spirits with which these frothy and boyling seeds abound, and are as instruments with which it begins to trace out the first lineaments of all the parts, to which afterwards (making use of the menstruous blood flowing to it) it gives in time growth, and the last perfection'.[22]

Attempts to prove the two seeds theory by anatomy — by locating the female ejaculatory vessels and so on — were obviously doomed to failure, but it fitted in well with people's subjective interpretation of sexual experience. According to this theory there were also plausible explanations as to how offspring resemble parents; how sex is determined; and how multiple births occur.

There was indeed a certain difference of opinion about the origin of the seed. Some thought women's seed and menstrual blood were one and the same thing; others thought that female seed, like male, came mostly from the brain, but a little also from each part of the body, otherwise all the parts would not be reproduced. It was generally agreed that seed could not come from the brain only, via the veins behind the ears and the spinal marrow, though Crooke claimed this ancient idea was the reason 'the common people thinke that the braines and marrow of the bones do engender much seede'. Some authors however continued to believe that cutting the veins behind the ears caused sterility. Crooke thought the idea that seed was drawn from every part of the body was 'a beggerly rudiment receiued from hand to hand among the Auncients'. In his opinion seed came from the testicles only, but spirits 'fall into the Testicles out of the whole body, and bring with them the Idea or forme of the parts and their formatiue faculty'.[23] Pechey reported that Glisson, Wharton and others thought a seedy juice passed along the nerve to the testicles, but 'Dr. *Willis* is of another Opinion; however the Seed must needs consist of a nervous Juice, and plenty of Spirits brought from the Brain, because of the great weakness, and enervation that is induced upon the Brain, and Nerves, by too great an use of Venery'.[24]

But probably the most widely held view was that some seed came from each part of the body: 'Certain it is, that all the Particles of the Seed, have a peculiar Determination, referring to that Part of the Body of the Parents, from whence they came, and which they are to form in the Child'.[25] Some thought children received the likeness of the parent 'by that *Quasi epilepsia in coitu* . . . by which is shook off from them [seeds] somewhat retaining the nature, and property of every part'.[26] Consequently, if parents had physical defects they passed them on to their children; this left unexplained however the hereditary nature of such defects, '*Deaf*, *Dumb*, *Blind*, *Mutilous*, produceing the like, (though such must also have been born so, else they beget Children as perfect as others)'.[27]

Sex was determined simply by which seed was stronger, or more plentiful. Men had both male and female seed, depending on which testicle it came from, but whether the same was true of female seed was not discussed. Naturally there were other factors, such as the force of imagination and the aspects of the planets, but that was so whichever theory of conception was believed to be correct.

McMath observed 'They will also have *Males* conceived in the *waxing* of the *Moon*, *Females* in the *waining* . . . many justly doubt any *Action* or *Rule* of the *Stars* upon things below'.[28] Mauriceau disbelieved this idea on the grounds of experience, having at the Hôtel Dieu on one and the same day delivered eleven women, all at their full time, of whom five had boys and six had girls.[29]

There were two possible reasons for multiple births; the most obvious and widely held was that the amount of seed ejaculated was unusually large, enough to form more than one embryo. This is the point of the story told by Mauriceau about a certain Mr Hebert, whose wife had four living children at a birth, and was asked by the Duke of Orleans '(in the presence of divers Persons of Quality) whether it were true, that he was so good a Fellow as to get his Wife with Child of those four at one bout? He answered very coldly, *Yes; and that he had certainly begat at the same time half a dozen, if his foot had not slipt*'.[30]

Alternatively, there might be a superfetation. Although normally the cervix was firmly closed after conception and the female seed voided by the imaginary by-pass vessels, on rare occasions a second conception might happen 'in the *Fervour* of a very *Libidinous Tickling Congress*, and a most ravening *Action* of the *Womb* for Generating; whence the *Womans Seed* may (in this *Warmth*, and *Vehemency*) Impetuously penetrate these *Passes*, and spring into the *Womb* . . . and the *Orifice* also (the *Womb* being thus wildly incited in this *Lustful Fervor*) may yet open in the *Sport* . . . for admitting the *Mans Seed* . . . against which let *Women* keep free of *Congress* their *First Months*'.[31]

Attempts were made to demonstrate whether twins were conceived on the same or separate occasions by noting whether they had one or two placentas, and were contained in the same or different membranes, though various observers came up with a range of conflicting answers. It was generally thought if there were separate membranes and two placentas there was probably a superfetation, if not, the twins were conceived on the same occasion. Mauriceau thought the relative rarity of separate placentas, which he put at ten in a 100 cases, showed how seldom superfetation happened. The accuracy of observation left something to be desired however; Mauriceau claimed to have seen boy and girl twins 'begotten at one and the same act of Copulation, as was manifest by their both having one and the same burthen'.[32] Some, with commendable caution, suggested these alleged single placentas might really be two fused together, and medical students in 1740 were shown an anatomical preparation of a twin placenta, one half injected with wax, the other left flaccid, to prove there was no connection between them.[33]

The ovum theory which gradually superseded the two seeds theory did not favour superfetation, and the ovists believed twins were caused by two eggs falling into the Fallopian tubes at once.

Before Harvey put forward the ovum theory he made numerous dissections of animals after copulation, mainly deer, and found no englobed ejaculate in the uterus. He decided therefore that the male seed did not form the embryo physically 'because it is certaine, that the *Geniture* of the *Male* doth not so much as reach to the *cavity* of the *Uterus*, much less abide there for any time; that *geniture* doth derive *foecundity* to the *Uterus* only by a kinde of *contagion* . . . by no *sensible corporeal Agent*'. This, he was careful to point out, was not a final statement, 'that so I may offer those things as true, which seem probable in such dark matters, until such time as they can be convinced of falsity or errour'. So he postulated an analogy between the conception of the mind and that of the uterus; 'Because, I say, there is no *Sensible thing* to be found in the *Uterus*, after coition; and yet there is a necessity, that something should be there, which may render the *female fruitful*; and that (in probability) can be no *corporeal essence*; we have no refuge left us, but to fly to meere *Conception*, and *reception* of *Species* without any matter; namely, to apprehend, that the same thing is effected in the *womb*, as in the *Braine*: unless some cunning *Philosopher*, whom the Gods have better provided for, can find out some *efficient cause*, which is not included in our recapitulation'.[34]

The cunning philosopher in question, Antoni van Leeuwenhoek, published his discovery of spermatozoa in 1677, but the discovery, although it solved Harvey's problem, attracted curiously little popular attention, and the only midwifery book to mention it at all refers to it as an abandoned idea. Rehearsing possible opinions about generation Dionis wrote: 'It is about ten Years since a new Opinion was broach'd, That Man, and all other Animals, proceeded from a Worm; and that there is an infinite number of little Worms in the Seed of every Animal, which they call'd *Seminary*, and which may be seen with the help of a Microscope'. This theory, he continued, was now out of favour because it meant only one worm impregnated the egg and many thousands were wasted.[35]

Pechey referred to the ovum theory in the earlier of his two books, though he still gave the older theory more prominence; 'Having made frequent mention of Womens Seed, I must here acquaint you that many Learned Physicians and Anatomists deny that Women have any Seed, for some Women send forth no humour as is called Seed, and yet they are Fruitful enough . . . 'Tis also said by some that a seminal Air or Vapour arising from the Mans Seed, and not the Seed it self causes Conception'.[36]

Dionis in the early eighteenth century found the ovum theory the more convincing. He thought the first two drops of male seed, that is to say the most spirituous, flew up into the ovarium and pierced the egg, which was passed back to the uterus by the Fallopian tube, stimulated by the volatile part of the seed going through. This explained how tubal pregnancy could arise, a relatively newly-observed phenomenon lending support to the ovum theory, which must formerly simply have caused sudden unexplained death. Pechey explained that the Fallopian tubes 'are the same in Women, that the horns of the womb are in other

Creatures . . . For as other Creatures always conceive in the Horns, so it has been sometimes observed, that a Conception has in a Woman bin contained in one of the tubes, which must have happened, when the Egg being received out of the stone into it, has been stopt in its passage to the womb'.[37] Twins, according to Dionis, always have separate membranes, whereas if they were formed from a mixture of two seeds all the conceptions would be included in one only.

The seminal vapour idea explained even better than the greedy womb how conception could occur without actual penetration. The causes of sterility now included 'An Obstruction of the *Tubae Fallopianae*, near to the Womb, which neither suffers the Seed to be carry'd up to the *Ovarium*, nor the *Ovum* to fall down into the Womb. The Structure of the Parts of the *Tuba* such, as hinders it embracing the *Ovum* straitly, to receive and convey it into the Womb. The Membrane of the *Ovarium* so thick, that the Seed cannot penetrate the *Ovum*, to loosen and bring it off'.[38]

In 1755 the ovum explanation of conception was received in *Aristotle's masterpiece*, though older ideas were still mentioned as true. Now however women's testicles 'contain nothing of Seed, as the Followers of *Galen* &c. erroneously imagine, yet they contain several Eggs . . . one of which being impregnated by the most spirituous Part of the Man's Seed in the Act of Coition, descends thro' the Oviducts into the Womb, where it is cherished till it becomes a live Child'.[39]

*Chapter Six*

# Development and Birth of the Foetus

Although considerable research and scientific speculation was devoted to embryology in the sixteenth and seventeenth centuries, it cannot be said that much real progress was made, partly because so many controversial hypotheses were advanced by academic writers, partly because it was not until the late-seventeenth century that the microscope came into use for such investigations. Embryology was thought to be the hardest part of anatomy, because it was difficult to observe. So far as the surgeon or midwife reading English textbooks only could know, some version of the ancient two seeds theory modified by modern writers, notably Coiter, was most likely to be accepted, at least until towards the turn of the eighteenth century.

Rueff may be taken as typical of the sixteenth century theory as it persisted in the seventeenth century also. According to him, on conception male and female seed curdled together in a mass, membranes promptly enclosed the mass and little fibres formed throughout, then three specks formed — the future brain, liver and heart. The outer layer of the brain-speck was baked and hardened by the heat of the womb into the skull, and from it nerves and sinews grew down the spine. Bones, cartilages and membranes were formed from seed, whereas flesh, heart, liver and lungs came from blood. The foetus was a milky blob for six days, then a blood-mass, then flesh, and by 18 days a fully-formed tiny human being.

According to Sharp the navel vein and then the liver formed first, and from them the venous system developed. Culpeper supplied a little more detail. After the amnion and chorion surrounded the seed, the navel vein developed, and piercing the membranes carried a drop of maternal blood to the seed, and from this blood the liver, vena cava and venous system developed. After that the great artery was formed, then the heart, and then the brain.

This account remained substantially the same at the end of the seventeenth century, in Barret's 1699 treatise for example.

Dr Chamberlain's version had a somewhat more complicated and detailed account, including the growth of the pulmonary artery to send the most purely concocted blood in the heart to the lungs, and the pulmonary vein 'to convey the cool aire from the bellows of the Lungs, to allay and temper the great heat of the heart'.[1]

According to Paré, after the formation of the blood vessels, the blood and vital spirit flowing to the congealed seed caused it to boil and ferment, and three bubbles formed — the liver from gross blood, the heart from spirituous blood and the brain from seed. Harvey, although he thought Coiter not altogether incompetent as an embryologist, dismissed 'his tale of the three globules' as a fable.[2] Nor did he think the liver was a mass of congealed blood from which more blood was made; he was convinced that blood came first, even before the heart which circulated it. Despite his own translated work however his theories about foetal development made no impact on the popular midwiferies, whereas the circulation of the blood and the ovum theory were both well represented by the turn of the eighteenth century.

It was generally believed in the sixteenth and seventeenth centuries that the formation time of boys and girls was different: 'Male children are engendered of a more hot and dry seed, and women of a more cold and moist: for there is much lesse strength in cold than in heat, and likewise in moisture than in drynesse; and that is the cause why it will be longer before a girle is formed in the womb than a boy'.[3] Mauriceau, as we have seen, denied this, on the grounds that 'Women are brought to Bed indifferently both of Sons and Daughters at the ordinary terme of nine months'. It was, he thought, *possible* to exceed the nine months, but generally such women were deceived in their reckoning. McMath agreed that by such mistakes some alleged five or six months births were really full term, 'And from the same mistake (or *Tricks* some may not avow) the *9th. Month Birth* is sometimes made the *7th.*'.[4]

The longer formation time of females was still asserted by Maubray however on the ancient grounds that the male, because of heat, 'arrives sooner to Perfection in *Formation* and *Animation*; and is consequently *sooner born* than the FEMALE, whose *Nature* is more *cold*, *flaccid*, and *weak*, even in the WOMB'.[5] Maubray thought most writers who made nine months the true time of gestation were mistaken: 'their fond Opinion seems not to be so much supported by any *Arguments* of *Natural Reason*, as by an *imaginary Experience*, founded upon *Hearsay*, or the *general Misconstruction* of WOMEN'. No less a man than Harvey moreover thought that gestation times of ten, eleven and even more months could exceptionally occur, and cited examples of such pregnancies.[6]

The matter was of practical importance, both to midwives to know whether to promote or retard labour, and to lawyers in matters of legitimacy and disputed inheritance. McMath noted 'some *Infants* may, and have been *Legittimatly Born* (and pronounced such) in the 12*th.* 13*th.* 14*th. Month* . . . Though yet such late *Births* are very justly suspected and observed almost ever in such *Widows* only, who for love of a dead *Husbands Fortune*, playes on after *Game*, and pretends him the Father of another mans *Child*: A *Trick* so frequent, as to make Clamorous, *Debates* among all *Courts* of *Justice* every where'.[7] In line with the uncertainty of the physicians, the legislators framing the Act relating to posthumous children's inheritance at the end of the seventeenth century declined to state any specific time after which a child could not be deemed legitimate.[8]

The matter of formation time and 'ensoulment' was also of much interest to theologians. Although the general belief was that the child was fully formed at 18 days, it was still not fully alive; it did not move, and its heart did not beat. At 45 days it 'obtained life', whatever that involved, but it did not quicken until 90 days. In sixteenth-century penitential practice 40 days was regarded as the time of ensoulment.[9] In the 1641 edition of Thomas Vicary's *The Englishman's treasure* 43 days was said to be the time of full perfection and receiving of the soul.

Uncertainty about the true length of gestation probably delayed the realisation that the longer the pregnancy advanced towards term the better the child was able to survive after birth. It was firmly believed by the ancients, and was still the general opinion of the world in Read's time, that an eight-month child could not survive, although a seven-month child could. Read himself disbelieved this idea: 'the first time that a Child may live when born, is the 7th Month compleat, and it may better from that time till the end of the 9th Month'.[10]

Most authors however continued to believe in the non-viability of the eight-month child, for which two explanations were given, one astrological, one physical. Paré mentioned both, but thought the physical one more likely: 'the reason thereof is, as the Astronomers suppose, because at that time Saturne ruleth, whose coldnesse and drynesse is contrary to the originall of life: but yet the physicall reason is more true; for the physitians say that the childe in the wombe doth often times in the seaventh moneth strive to bee set at liberty', thus weakening itself so that unless it was successfully born then, it was too enfeebled to survive the birth until another month elapsed.[11] Culpeper had his own eccentric explanation for the superior life-expectation of the seven-month child. It was due, he said, to the perfection of the number seven, 'which if I were but writing Divinity, I could prove by Scripture to be the perfectest number that is'.

It seems possible that on this subject popular opinion was ahead of the textbooks, or of Maubray at least. He thought the planets and the perfection of the number seven had a lot to do with it, but the real reason why an eight-month child could not survive was its endeavours to be born the month before, 'tho' I have heard some loquacious *Women* strenuously aver the *contrary*'.[12] Maubray however had a genius for supporting the wrong hypothesis, and most writers in the eighteenth century do not refer to the subject, evidently because it was no longer accepted.

We have seen that the two seeds theory adequately explained hereditary likeness and deformities, but the ovum theory was somewhat less satisfactory in this respect. The ovists tended to support the very old idea that the power of the mother's imagination imprinted the likeness of one or other parent, or even of more distant relatives, on the foetus. Mauriceau, though not an ovist, inclined to this view. He mentioned the case of a lady who had twins, one like her husband, the other like her lover. Although Mauriceau was disposed to think that this was a case of superfetation, it did not altogether prove that theory because imagination might have caused the same effect.[13] But Mauriceau thought the influence of imagination was limited to the time of conception, and thus those who thought birth marks were caused by the mother's longing to drink red wine were wrong; they were really caused by some extravasated blood, at the time the infant was formed. He also said his own arrival in the world marked with a few smallpox, was not because of his mother thinking about his elder brother, then dying of the disease, but from the contagious air she breathed while nursing his brother, which affected him in utero through the mass of her blood.[14]

But Mauriceau was almost alone in thinking the power of imagination to be relatively unimportant. Authors quoted well-known examples, such as the queen of Ethiopia who bore a white child from thinking about 'a marvellous white thing' when she lay with the king. Or of the woman who, conversely, at the time of conception beholding the picture of a blackamoor, conceived and brought forth a black child. The case of the gentlewoman in Suffolk whose face was spotted with blood passing her butcher's, and had a child similarly marked was another example. Sharp said in general 'sometimes the mother is frighted or conceives wonders, or longs strangely for things not to be had, and the child is markt accordingly by it'.

There was after all proof of the effect of imagination in Scripture: 'Imagination is powerful in all living creatures, for by it *Jacob's* Ewes conceived spotted, and grisled, the peeled rods being set before them when they were in conjunction'.[15] With so much 'proof' of the effect of imagination Mauriceau probably had little success in urging women to 'wean themselves from these vain apprehensions, which they say they have to such things (every moment) and serves some of them for a pretext to cover their liquorishness'. Certainly the 1755 *Aristotle's masterpiece* quoted Jacob's sheep and the gentlewoman spotted with blood at the butcher's as good evidence, and in 1773 the obstetrician John Leake said stories of the effect of imagination, such as the speckled cattle in Genesis, were still too readily believed.[16]

We may note briefly that monstrous births were thought to be caused by imagination, or by improper congress at the time of menstruation, or unnatural copulation with beasts. The question of devils engendering with human beings, though quite seriously debated, will be taken up in a later chapter, but even less 'evidence' seems to have been invoked in this matter than the dubious coincidences which supported the imagination theory.

Anatomists were very divided over the number and purpose of the membranes round the foetus, a difference of opinion made more confusing by lack of agreement about the terms with which to describe them. At first it was thought that the placenta was a membrane, albeit a fleshy one, and the infant broke through it as well as the other membranes, at birth. According to Raynald the placenta, which he called 'chorion', did not enclose the whole body but girdled it round the middle, and was joined to the womb by veins: 'Agayne the substaunce of this Choryon is not thyn lyke a skyn, bladdar or caule, but of all other parts of the boody, it may be most wurthelye resemblyd to the splene or melt in a man or best. The corpulencye or thycknesse whereof is as muche or more as the thyckenesse of the thumbe. The couloure swartisshe blacke'.[17] Later authors accepting this description called it the 'hoop-caul'.

Sharp attributed this confusion of chorion and placenta to the anatomist Columbus. Vesalius did not think the placenta was a membrane, but the illustrations in the 1543 *Fabrica* show it as Raynald described it, whereas those in the 1555 version are much more accurate.[18] Paré thought it was a membrane, but formed from the cotyledons, which 'swell up in women, and are like a rude piece of flesh of a finger and a halfe thicke; which begirt all the naturall parts of the infant shut up in the wombe'. Even as late as the 1682 *The English midwife enlarged* the confusion of chorion and placenta persisted, although by the late-seventeenth century the placenta had generally ceased to be regarded as a membrane.

There was also considerable argument over the other membranes, some following the ancients and asserting that there was a membrane called allantoides, as well as the chorion and amnion, others denying the existence of this membrane. Those who believed it existed thought its function was to contain foetal urine, whereas the amnion contained foetal sweat. Those who denied its existence held that the amnion contained both sweat and urine. Paré described the careful methods of dissection he had used without success to find it, and concluded there was no such membrane, but that the ancients who wrote otherwise wrote from observations made in beasts.[19] Mauriceau did not believe in this membrane either, but there was still no complete agreement: 'Most Authors are so dark in the descriptions they make of these Membranes, that it is very hard to conceive them as they are, by the explication they make of them. They do not so much as agree in the number of them, some account three as well for a Child as a Beast, to wit, the *Chorion*, the *Amnios*, and the *Allantoides*; others account but two, because there is no *Allantoides* in a humane *Fœtus*'.[20]

There was equal disagreement about the existence or not of the urachus. Paré and Mauriceau, who rightly denied the existence of the membrane allantoides, wrongly denied the existence of the urachus. Paré could not find it at all; Mauriceau said it existed, but that it was not a vessel, but only a ligament. Those who thought that there was an allantoides tended also to believe that the urachus conveyed foetal urine either into it, or to the mother's bladder. Presumably the question arose, in a period when embryonic material for dissection was hard to come by, from failing to distinguish between the structure at different stages of development.

By the early-eighteenth century authors had stopped including embryology in the midwifery books, and these matters were quietly dropped, though Willughby justly pointed out that if midwives understood about the membranes they could not, as many did, imagine the child could stick to the mother's back.

The discussion of the membranes and placenta was naturally much involved with notions about foetal nutrition, excretion and respiration, which were also very varied. In addition to the idea that the amniotic fluid was a mixture of foetal sweat and urine there was a suggestion put forward by Mauriceau that the water was caused by transpiration. Paré, who thought it was excrementitious, said it had mainly a cushioning and supportive function. Harvey however denied it was excrementitious, and thought it was nutritive. This was a variant on the Hippocratic idea that the child sucked blood from the placenta for nourishment, a notion which claimed support from the presence of the sucking reflex at birth, and of meconium in the intestines. Crooke, rejecting the idea that the infant was nourished by mouth excused Hippocrates this error 'because in those times the skill of Anatomy was but in the infancie; or else we may think that this, as many other things, was foysted into his worke'. Culpeper was voicing the opinion of the majority however in claiming that all modern writers agreed that the child received its nourishment by the navel. He was also expressing a majority opinion, though not a unanimous one, when he said it was nourished in the womb by menstrual blood, and after birth also by menstrual blood turned into milk.

The whole subject of menstruation was much debated, and the debate was still active at the end of the time under consideration. The twin ideas that menstruation was a sort of natural blood-letting or purgation necessary for health, and that it had a formative or nutritive function in pregnancy were both very ancient, and both still accepted in a relatively unsophisticated way in the sixteenth century.

According to the purgation interpretation, menstruation was needed for the health of women, but not of men. Men's greater heat enabled them to digest their food completely, whereas women could not, so that something remained on their liver after each meal, which was periodically accumulated and rejected by the body. On the other hand menstruation was essential for conception. Pechey at the end of the seventeenth century combined both ideas in this statement: '*Menstruous blood* is nothing else but an *Excrement* of the third concoction, gathered together every Month, and purged out. Which Purgation being duly made, the Woman is then in perfect health of body; but if they come not down according to their accustomed times, and seasons, or do not come down at all, the Woman neither can conceive nor engender'.[21]

Although some modern writers assigned venemous properties to menstrual blood after the style of Pliny, this view was not accepted by many authorities in the sixteenth century. Even in the fifteenth century it was held that the infant was fed with menstrual blood. Sharp refuted the opinion of modern writers such as Columbus and Fernelius who denied the infant could be fed with menstrual blood, 'because such blood is impure, and will, where it falls, destroy Plants, and Trees, Dogs will run mad that eat it, and ofttimes hurts the women themselves . . . this then were ill food for a tender infant. But to answer all: If the woman be in good health, her monthly courses are no bad blood for quality though they hurt in quantity being more than she can concoct'.[22]

Raynald considered the menstrual blood was designed to nourish the foetus, and simply evacuated as unprofitable when there was no pregnancy. He also pointed out that a woman who did not menstruate could not have children, because although she might conceive, there would be no nutriment for the child to grow. It was in his view an error to call menstruation a purgation 'for vndoutedly this blud is euen as pure and holsu*m* as all the rest of the blud'; the stories of Albertus Magnus and others about the venemous nature of menstrual blood were 'but dreames and playne dotage'.[23]

But a medical student of 1740 noted that although such notions had been 'abollish'd since ye circulation of the Blood have been made appear, yet in some countrys in England ye notion of its being contagious is retained still among ye Vulgar'.[24] It was doubtless one of the vulgar who once owned my copy of the *Aristotle* books, on a blank page of which is written in a rough hand 'One hair of a woman's Cunt when her flowers are upon her put it in Dung will breed a Serpent'.

Sadler thought the menstrual blood was in itself pure, but those who thought it venemous were not entirely wrong, because it might acquire ill qualities and become corrupt by the admixture of vicious humours, or by staying too long in the uterus, and in that sense Pliny, Fernelius and the rest who thought it poisonous were to be understood. Nevertheless it continued to be believed that children conceived during menstruation would be sickly, leprous or defective, or at least subject to plethoric diseases.

Although Raynald denied it, the notion that menstruation had something to do with the phases of the moon also persisted late on in the time under consideration. According to McMath it should break out 'mostly about the presence of the *Moon*, (which some make the *Cause* of this *Periodick* appearance . . . )'. Pechey thought the different phases of the moon caused women in different age groups to menstruate at different times in the month. Dr Chamberlain observed that young women had courses mostly at the new moon, older ones at the full. This was deemed very useful to know when prescribing medicine 'when the Courses are stop'd, and they know not well the time when their evacuation should be'. Suppression of the courses was usually caused by the blood sticking in the veins, and the flow to the womb obviously needed to be provoked by blood-letting in the foot.

Suppression of the courses was viewed with much more concern than their excessive flow. This latter was generally caused by the admixture of vicious humours which ought to be allowed to flow away, unless the woman was noticeably weakened. Since the normal menstrual flow was put at somewhere between one and two pints 'excessive' flow must have been quite rare. But the whole notion of quantification in physiology was new and unfamiliar. In the first work devoted entirely to menstruation Freind assumed the infant to be fed by the blood otherwise lost in menstruation, and 'proved' it working on a 20 ozs monthly flow and an average birth weight of 12 lbs. He did admit however many infants were lighter than this.[25] He considered the flow was due to the weight of accumulated blood combined with the upright posture peculiar to human beings, and broke out when the pressure ruptured the capillaries, both in the uterus and vagina.[26] He also stated that whether the blood was arterial or venous it did not come from the larger vessels, as earlier writers had thought. Bartholin for instance said 'Menstrual blood is shed forth by the Arteries in Women not with Child ... the colour of the Menstrual blood in healthy women, declares that it is Arterial blood'.[27]

According to Paré 'The suppressed or stopped tearms in women that are great with childe, are divided into three parts: the more pure portion maketh the nutriment for the childe, the second ascendeth by little and little into the dugs, and the impurest of all remaineth in the womb about the infant, and maketh the secundine or after-birth'.[28] Maubray explained that vomiting occurred in early pregnancy because the foetus being too small to need it all, part of the blood turned into putrid humours, whereas later it needed the whole of the menstruous blood for nutriment.

It was assumed by most authors that menstrual blood and breast milk were essentially the same fluid, but a change of colour occurred.[29] Paré considered it a great dispensation of nature that the blood turned white, otherwise people would be shocked by 'so grievous and terrible a spectacle of the childes mouth so imbrued and besmeared with blood'.[30] Dr Chamberlain quoted a case reported by Brassavolus of a woman 'out of whose Breasts, issued bloud, instead of milk; which may well be: For Nurses have their Courses stopt, because the bloud doth return from the womb unto the Breasts, and is by them concocted, and turned into milk . . . but in this example, the bloud came out crude, and unconcocted, or unturned'.[31]

Rueff and other early authors claimed there were two veins from the breasts to the womb by which the blood ascended to be turned into milk. But Willis said 'it is greatly disputed among Authors, by what Ductus's that Humour is conveyed both unto the Breast, and unto the *Placenta*'. He explained that some thought milk was engendered from blood freely concocted in the glands, others that chyle went to both breasts and uterus from the viscera, through occult passages, without any alteration. He personally thought a portion of chyle made in the stomach was absorbed into the bloodstream, 'which having gotten the Vehicle of the Blood, and being brought by the Arteries into the Glands destinated here and there for receiving it before it is assimilated, and being separated, is depos'd again from the Mass of Blood'. Thus the infant was fed in the womb by 'Milk, or a nourishable Humour . . . deposed in a great Plenty about the *Placenta* of the Womb: but, after Delivery, that long Suppression of the *Menses* is recompenc'd by a copious flowing of the *Lochia*, and the Milk, within three days space, leaving wholly the Womb, flies plentifully into the Breasts . . . and if the Milk be driven from the Breasts, it restagnates again towards the Womb, and is voided forth together with the *Lochia* under the form of a whitish Humour'.[32]

Harvey said women called it 'the coming of the *Milke*, when their *purgations* are now no longer died with *blood*'.[33] Mauriceau also said that the lochia, after the blood ceased to be mingled with them, 'do almost resemble, in colour and consistence, troubled Milk, which makes the World believe it is Breast Milk which is in that manner emptied downwards; but in truth it is an Abuse as great as common'.[34]

By the end of the seventeenth century the two veins passing between the breasts and the womb by which the blood and milk changed places had, not surprisingly, still not been found, but it was not a concept as yet wholly abandoned. Portal, who still believed that when the milk was repelled from the breasts it was discharged with the lochia, was also still hoping to discover this mythical channel: 'nature has certain hidden channels not discoverable by our eyes. The same may be said of turning, or the motion of the milk in women in child-bed . . . Mr. Briset and I have in our hospitals of Paris open'd a good number of dead bodies of child-bed women, but could never as yet discover any passage whereby the milk might pass to the womb'.[35]

Just as some authors thought the breast-milk was really menstrual blood in the breasts, others thought the menstrual blood turned to milk in the womb, and so the infant was fed with breast-milk before as well as after birth. Thus if a woman had her courses during pregnancy or had much milk in her breasts it was evident the child was in danger, and not strong enough to take the nourishment.

Most authors believed pregnant women had milk in their breasts long before the birth: 'women with Child about the fourth moneth have their Breasts swoln with milk . . . so soon as the infant moves there is Milk bred in the Breasts as any one may prove that will'.[36] But Harvey said the milk was not found in quantity before the seventh month, and Mauriceau that it was not proper milk, but a wheyish substance, and neither thick nor very white, until after labour when the mother began to suckle her child.

Some authors thought women who had never been pregnant could have milk in their breasts. According to Paré this happened to marriageable virgins who were full of juice and seed, and they had as much milk as nurses. Crooke said 'It was disputed of old, and is yet a question amongst the multitude, whether Milke can be engendred in a womans breasts before she haue had the company of man and conceyued'.[37] McMath thought that there were such cases: '*Lascivious Virgins*, and *Widows* wholly intent to Lustful *Cogitations*, and much in thinking of *Breasts*, *Milk*, and their Sucking, wantonly rubbing, tickling, or Sucking thereof, may have got *Milk* in them . . . yet that is most rare'.[38] So as late as 1755 it was claimed that virgins might have a sort of milk in their breasts made of blood that could not get out of the womb and so went to the breasts.[39]

We have seen that the placenta was thought at first to be a membrane, made of the dregs of menstrual blood. Paré thought it formed a sort of bed for the child to lie in, and Sharp, in 1671, that it was chiefly to support the child, though by then most anatomists thought it had more important uses. Mauriceau considered its chief function was to purify the maternal blood, which was never good during pregnancy, and fit it for the foetus. Harvey thought it prepared blood in a way similar to the liver and the breasts, and that its chief function was therefore nutritive. Commonly English writers called it the 'womb-liver' referring to this function. Mauriceau and Pechey were the only authors who seem to have thought the maternal and foetal bloodstreams did not actually flow into each other.[40] Dionis indeed clearly thought they were directly connected: 'When a Woman is with Child, the Arteries open into the *Placenta*, from which, by the Navel-String, the *maternal* Blood is carry'd to the *Foetus*, for its

Nourishment; and the remainder of this Blood is brought back to the *Placenta*, which discharges it into the Mouths of the Veins, to be carry'd back to the Mass of Blood'.[41] He denied Mauriceau's view that blood passed by 'natural transfusion' into the placenta, and then into the infant's own circulatory system, the foetal venous blood returning again to the placenta to be 'elaborated' and circulated once more.[42] He considered the placenta did not purify and elaborate blood, which could only be done by the heart.

Pechey however said that 'Spirituous blood is driven from the Child by the beating of its Heart to the Womb-cake, and the Membranes for their nourishment, from which, what blood remains circulates back again in the umbilical vein, together with the nutritious juice afresh imbibed by the Capillaries dispersed in the Womb-cake; but Blood and Vital Spirits are not carried by the Arteries from the Mother to the Child, as *Galen* and many others have taught'.[43]

Mauriceau also thought the placenta performed the functions of respiration for the infant. Noting that obstruction of the circulation in the umbilical cord caused rapid foetal death, although the infant's own circulation was not impeded, he concluded ' 'tis either absolutely necessary that the Blood, for want of respiration, should be elaborated or prepared in the *Placenta*, and therefore there must be a free communication, or for want of it, that the Infant must immediately breath by the mouth'.[44]

Even Raynald, though his concepts were less sophisticated, thought that two arteries passed into the child, and 'throughe these artyres liuely spirite, & fresshe aere, is diriuied out of the mother into the childe, wherwith the naturall hete of the chylde is viuified and refresshed'.[45] Paré also, who did not think the child's heart beat, believed it respired by the motion of the spirituous blood in the arteries. McMath, denying that the infant breathed by mouth, as those who told stories of infants crying in the womb supposed, pointed out that the outward air could have no access, except by 'an *Airy* Substance, or *Nitro-aereous Particles* the nourishing *Juyces* comes filled with'.[46]

One interesting reflection of these ideas was seen in the conduct of post-mortem caesarean section. Although Paré knew that once the mother's lungs stopped moving the infant could receive no more air, and Guillemeau after him that the child respired only through the mother, yet Guillemeau and even later authors recommended holding the mother's mouth and genitals open to help prevent the child suffocating. But Read stated categorically that this was useless, though it might be prudent to keep up the practice because of the expectations of the bystanders, who might otherwise think the surgeon negligent should the child be found dead.

The causes given for the onset of normal labour at term, as might be expected, were mainly derived from the supposed wants of the foetus. The importance of the foetus and the uterine action in the birth process was also variously assessed, and most, especially earlier, authors held that the foetus effected its own egress while others believed that it played little part.

We have already seen that the foetus was for a long time believed to turn and make an attempt to be born in the seventh month. Read agreed that it usually turned head down at that time, but the reason was that the head and upper parts had grown heavier and thus fell downwards. But he knew that some infants turn later, some not at all. The foetus was generally depicted in the breech position, though to illustrate various malpresentations early texts showed it looking about three years old, arms and legs impossibly extended.

Verbal descriptions of the foetal position, albeit as a breech, were rather more accurate, and remained remarkably constant from Raynald to Pechey: 'the Infant lies with his Back and his Buttocks leaning against the Back of the Mother, the head inclined, and touching his Breast with his Chin: resting his two Hands upon his Knees; his *Navel* and his *Nose* between his two *Knees*, with his two *Eyes* upon his two *Thumbs*, his *Legs* folded backward, and touching his *Buttocks* with each *Leg*'.[47]

The turning attributed by Read to weight was thought by other authors to be caused by the infant seeking for the outward air, or finding itself cramped and seeking release, or being driven by the insufficiency of the food supply to seek an alternative. The infant was seen as active in labour, almost consciously so. If it were strong the labour went well, if weak it was difficult. Cases of infants being born spontaneously after the mother's death were reported, and attributed, together with cases of ruptured uterus, to the infant's violent efforts. It was thought that the infant itself broke through the membranes, and where it was weak it needed help. Even Willughby, who knew that the uterus did most of the work, thought the infant struggled to break the membranes.

Harvey described the birth overnight of a foal to an infibulated white mare belonging to the queen, which was found in the morning with its haunch torn open and the foal beside it; but Harvey, partly misled by a false comparison with chickens breaking out of the shell, thought this proved the incredible force of the young foal, and not of the uterine action.[48]

Even where the uterus was credited with a part in the proceedings it was thought the kicking of the foetus was needful to stimulate uterine action. Wolveridge wrote 'the true pains of a woman in travail . . . are nothing else but the force of the infant now perfect'. According to McMath uterine inertia was caused by the infant ceasing to move and to kick, and so late as 1724 Maubray believed that the infant's efforts to be born drew the uterus into action by consent.

It had however not escaped the notice of writers even at an early date that dead babies did somehow get born. Raynald attributed this expulsion to the muscles of the abdomen and midriff. Harvey thought that the dead birth gave off acrimonious humours which stimulated the uterus to relieve itself. Dr Chamberlain however said clearly that in every case the uterine muscles expel the foetus. And Mauriceau wrote, 'if they that practise Deliveries, make a true reflection on it, they will find, that it is the Matrix alone, assisted with the compression of the muscles of the lower Belly and *Diaphragma*, which cause the expulsion of the Child, being stirred up by its weight, and not able to be further extended to contain it; and not, as is ordinarily believed, that the Infant (being no longer able to stay there for want of the nourishment and refreshment) useth his pretended indeavours to com forth thence, and to that purpose kicking strongly, he breaks with his feet the membranes'.[49] But even in 1773, long after Smellie's work on the mechanism of labour had established the passivity of the foetus, Leake noted that the infant 'does not usually struggle in the birth, as generally thought'.

Yet another fallacy about the labour process abandoned in this period, though not without a struggle, was the idea that the bones of the pelvis separated during labour to let the foetus pass.

Paré stated that he had opened the bodies of women who died in childbirth, in whom he found the ilium and sacrum separated. Willughby, quoting Harvey, accepted that 'the fore-said bones do easily give way to the parting Infant; and by gaping open, do amplifie the whole region of the Hypogastrium or lower belly', yet he admitted he had never seen it in his own practice.[50]

This viewpoint was modified by later writers, some saying this separation was not really normal, and occurred only in difficult labours, others that the bones did not actually separate, but the connecting ligaments softened and stretched. Mauriceau thought nothing of the sort happened. Paré, he said, was mistaken in attributing the separation of the bones observed by him in an executed subject to her recent labour, it was more likely due to the fall from the scaffold or some other injury. Women at the Hôtel Dieu were often delivered some distance from the recovery wards and walked there very well, which they could not do if their pelvis were disjointed. And as to the ligaments being moistened by humours from the womb, this was 'as far from Truth as Reason; for Anatomy convinceth us clearly, that the Womb by no means toucheth these places, whereby to mollifie them by its humours; as also, that these bones are so joyned by the cartilage, that it is very difficult to separate them with a Knife'. The female pelvis, Mauriceau maintained, being larger and shaped differently from the male, only presents an obstacle to the birth in deformed persons.[51]

The process of involution was not much regarded until the end of our period, although early writers were much concerned that the lochia should flow duly, by which they meant copiously. It was originally thought that the lochia consisted of the residue of exhausted menstrual blood and vicious humours accumulated during pregnancy while the womb was closed, and this view was still partly current at the end of the seventeenth century. Since the normal menses were supposed to be a pint and a half, the lochia should be a pint or three quarters of a pint daily, diminishing gradually for 30 days after the birth of a boy, and 40 after a girl. The sayings of nurses who urged their patients to eat well and make up the lost blood were dismissed as mere fooleries due to their ignorance that the blood lost 'is but unnecessary and useless Blood, dam'd up in the Womb for the space of nine Months; the Efflux of which, must needs be conducive to Health'.[52]

Mauriceau however denied the lochia represented the relics of the infant's nourishment, and said the blood was the very same with all the rest in the body. He thought that the flow was simply caused by the wound of the placental site gradually healing.[53] It was slowly realised that the womb itself stopped the bleeding by contraction, and by the end of our period Giffard had actually observed this happening: 'Passing my Hand a second time, I found the Uterus very much contracted and collapsed, so that I could not easily turn my Hand in it; by which it appears how soon the Uterus endeavours to regain its natural state.'[54]

*Chapter Seven*

# Diagnosis of Pregnancy and Ante-natal Regimen

The accurate diagnosis of pregnancy was until very recently a most intractable problem. On the one hand many tests and signs had been suggested, and believed in, from very ancient times, but on the other hand experience showed that none of them could be implicitly relied on. The problem was particularly pressing where the woman was on trial for her life, and where she was thought to be in need of medical treatment, such as bleeding in the foot, which would be contra-indicated by pregnancy.

The difficulties thus encountered by conscientious practitioners were emphasised by the more responsible authors, but large numbers of midwives and empirics, and not a few authors, confidently claimed to be able to tell not only if a woman was pregnant, but also whether the child would be a boy or a girl.

Among the many signs of pregnancy described, the cessation of the menses was not considered particularly important, at least by earlier authors. As we have seen, the nature of the menstrual flow was not understood, and since in practice women do sometimes menstruate in early pregnancy and mistake their dates, now as then, perhaps the lack of emphasis on this sign is not surprising.

The persistence throughout the period of signs and tests of ancient origin and no value is to be explained partly by lack of certainty in the matter on a scientific level, and partly by the assumption of knowledge in such matters by women themselves, most of whose ideas were traditional.

Most of the practitioner authors advised great circumspection, whether in a judicial or a private case, in giving a professional opinion about conception. Pechey pointed out that many of the signs of pregnancy occurred also in a 'suppression of the courses, and none of them are so very certain, as not sometimes to fail us; wherefore in trials of Women, and upon giving physick to them, great caution must be used; for after the Execution of some Women, they have been found with

Child contrary to the judgment of the Midwifes, and others after a long course of Physick to open obstructions, and to cure a Dropsie, have been delivered of Children'.[1] Sharp declared that women themselves, especially young ones of their first child, 'are so ignorant commonly, that they cannot tell whether they have conceived or not, and not one of twenty almost keeps a just account, else they would be better provided against the time of their lying in, and not so suddenly be surprised as many of them are'.[2]

This did not happen only to young and ill-educated women; Mauriceau mentioned the wife of a counsellor of the court 'who after having been in a course of Physick of six or seven whole months for the Dropsie, under an eminent Physician, was at length brought to bed of a Child'.[3] Another lady, feeling ill and thinking she was not pregnant, persuaded her physican to bleed and purge her, whereupon she miscarried at three months.

Midwives and men-midwives alike made these mistakes. In a case of vaginal closure operated on by Guillemeau the patient was nevertheless pregnant, but a midwife told her husband 'that there was no likelihood, nay it was impossible to thinke that a yong woman of eighteene yeares of age should be with child, her husband hauing neuer entred within her maiden cloister: and that with threshing onely at the barne doore, she could not be full'.[4] In another case Portal and others judged a woman not pregnant, because the cervix was not tightly closed and she had her menses, but when she died of a fever she was found at autopsy four months gone.

During the time in question however, the numerous alleged signs given by earlier authors were gradually dropped, and by the beginning of the eighteenth century had been whittled down to a few which we would still regard as useful. Date alone however is not a reliable guide to what signs were believed in. Raynald for example showed a healthy scepticism, and after mentioning various ancient signs he warned that 'these toke*n*s, although they haue a certayn reason, & apparence, yet be they not alwayes vnfallyble, but onely lycklye'.[5] But a century later Culpeper confidently stated that if the vein under the eye was discoloured, and the woman neither menstruating nor overtired 'you may certainly conclude her to be with child . . . I have told many Women of it before they have been with child a fortnight and never failed'.[6]

Many of the old signs and tests were still being trotted out in *Aristotle's masterpiece*; these signs included fullness and milk in the breasts; strange longings and depraved appetites; veins under the tongue being greenish; veins in the neck swollen; the cervix tightly closed; and many others.

Although Guillemeau thought it impossible to tell whether the child would be a boy or a girl he nevertheless listed the signs commonly believed in. These were largely based on the equation of males and the right side, females and the left; thus one breast would be fuller and firmer than the other, one eye brighter, one side of the belly more prominent, and the woman would step first with the foot corresponding to the side the child lay on. Women were also alleged to be much healthier, better coloured and more cheerful if the child was a boy, sickly pregnancies usually producing a girl.

This sort of sex diagnosis was clearly much demanded by women, 'which is absolutely impossible; though there is hardly a Midwife which will not boast her self able to resolve it'.[7] Even in the eighteenth century Dionis advised the surgeon, hard pressed to foretell the child's sex, to fall back on the widely-believed Hippocratic signs, despite their total lack of foundation. *Aristotle's experienced midwife* still listed the signs, which however were 'not all to be trusted, yet there is some Truth among 'em'.

Uroscopy, though it had fallen into much disrepute since the middle ages, when it was believed almost anything could be diagnosed from the urine, was still in popular use for pregnancy diagnosis. It was said that in pregnant women 'The Urine becomes White, with a Cloud swimming at the top, wherein are to be seen many Atomes; which in the first Month do commonly sink to the bottom; and if ye shake it, it seems like Wool'.[8]

But uroscopy was viewed as scientifically dubious by many authors; Sudell argued 'I know it is common . . . for women to send their waters to the Doctors on purpose. But that neither the sex nor gravidity can be discerned and discovered barely by the urine, I will demonstrate'. Its supporters were the ordinary women: 'I know many will say I have carried mine and others waters, and such and such a Doctor hath told me right, and he can tell', but in Sudell's view this was mere luck.[9]

There were also various urine tests for pregnancy; for example: 'Take also the Urine of a Woman, and put it in a bason a whole night together, with a clean and bright needle in it, if the woman have conceived, the needle will be scattered full of red speckles, but if not, it will be black and rusty'.[10] Or if the urine was stopped up in a glass three days and then had small living creatures in it, the woman had conceived, 'For the Urin, which was before Part of her own Substance, will be generative as well as its mistress'.[11] Bran, nettles, sage leaves and so on could be steeped in urine and the results noted. Such tests were still supported by *Aristotle's masterpiece*.

It seems likely that authors often included the old tests and signs in deference to popular belief. Some tests however were still given credence; it was still thought diagnostic of pregnancy if the cervix was tightly closed. This test was not particularly helpful in diagnosing early pregnancy, but men-midwives accustomed to such examinations learned to tell the nearness of pregnancy to term by the degree of cervical uptake. This was important where premature labour pains occurred, and also, as Mauriceau pointed out, in the admission of women at the Hôtel Dieu, many of whom presented themselves for admission long before they were due, to get free board and lodging.

By the eighteenth century, although the old signs survived in popular literature, in the practice of experienced surgeons the signs of pregnancy were very similar to those relied on until the present century, namely the size of the abdomen, fullness of the breasts, darkening of the areola, followed by nausea in some cases, and perceptible foetal movement. Cessation of menstruation was now regarded as the most important sign.

The regimen to be followed once pregnancy was diagnosed was based on the right use of the classical six 'non-naturals', air, food and drink, exercise and rest, sleep and waking, fullness and emptiness, and passions of the mind. Barret claimed the right ordering of these things would keep the pregnant woman in good frame, unlike those fine ladies who by cossetting themselves were 'frequently out of Tune, always stuffing their Guts with slops, having their Chamber Windows adorn'd like an Apothecaries Shop with Pill-Boxes and Gally-Pots'.[12]

The correction of disorders if they arose was also necessary, and professional ante-natal care was virtually limited to this. Jonas advised those who had any disease about the genitals 'to be loked vnto and cured before the tyme of labor commethe, by the aduyse of some experte Surgion'. It was not common to seek professional confirmation of the pregnancy itself until the eighteenth century, and then only among the upper social classes, but most books added advice on ante-natal regimen to the do-it-yourself pregnancy tests. The first thing was to bespeak a good midwife, preferably one who had herself borne many children. Lamenting the general lack of spiritual preparation for childbirth one author considered the usual preparation to be entirely practical: 'linnen and other necessaryes for the child, a nurse, a midwife, entertainment for the women that are called to their labour, a warm convenient chamber, &c.'[13]

A mass of advice was given however to ensure health and prevent miscarriage. Pregnant women ought not to live in dirty narrow lanes or near common dunghills, lest the bad smells caused miscarriage. Sudden loud noises, as of thunder, artillery, and great bells, were dangerous for the same reason. Riding on horseback, in coaches or waggons might jolt the child and cause miscarriage, but it was safe to take a sedan or litter. The best sort of exercise was gentle walking in low-heeled shoes, because 'big bellied Women are apt to stumble, because they cannot see their feet'. The arms could be exercised in carding or spinning, but care must be taken not to strain the ligaments of the womb by stretching upwards, the woman ought therefore not to dress her own head.

Most midwives and authors advised women to exercise more near the time of delivery, but Mauriceau disagreed and thought this bad advice was a great cause of hard labour, since if 'instead of giving her self rest, she falls a jumping, walking, running up and down stairs' and so forth, the child would very likely turn sideways or in some other wrong posture.

Sleeping after dinner was bad for pregnant women, 'but in the morning they may take their ease; yet not turning (as some Ladies do) the night into day, and the day into night, too frequently now made use of'.[14] It was generally known that city dames who lived lives of idle luxury had fewer children than labouring country women, and those they had were sicklier.

Hygiene was largely ignored, though Raynald thought washing the hair every ten days did no harm, providing it was well dried afterwards with hot cloths. But bathing, especially in the common hot houses, he did not encourage. La Vauguion indeed stated categorically that a pregnant woman must never bath for fear the womb opened.

All authors united to condemn strait-lacing and stiff whalebone busks, which caused injury to the breasts, stunted and deformed the child's growth, and made the belly after childbirth wrinkled and pendent. But supporting the belly with a swathe-band, and anointing it with pomatum would keep it smooth 'and from hanging down like a tripe'. A little ingot of steel worn between the breasts would keep them from growing too big and stop the milk curdling.

It was generally thought sexual intercourse was inadvisable, at least in the first few months, for fear of shaking the child and bringing down the courses.[15] Some authors thought intercourse in the ninth month however would 'help and hasten the deliuery . . . for comming into the world after this acte, he is commonly enwrapped and compassed with slime, which helpeth his comming forth'.[16]

Sharp noted that women are almost alone among female creatures in desiring copulation after conception, but that it was needful for man that it should be so, because polygamy is forbidden by the laws of God. Culpeper thought it impractical to forbid copulation during pregnancy, 'for I know well enough the Nature of Man is so vicious, that he must have to do with his Wife, or some body else in that time, or do that which is worse than either'. Still, it was generally agreed that intercourse was not safe unless very moderate, for it was well known that 'common Whores (who often use Copulation) have never, or very rarely any Children; For the Grass seldom grows in a Path that is commonly trodden in'.[17]

Bleeding and purging, or at least clysters, during pregnancy, occasioned some difference of opinion. It was most important to prevent costiveness, and some authors approved of clysters for the purpose; according to Rueff this would not cause abortion, as the unskilful believed. Willughby approved of clysters, as did most authors, at the end of pregnancy, but Guillemeau and others thought pregnant women in the early months should avoid clysters if at all possible.

Bleeding was also the subject of disagreement. Although bleeding, in the foot especially, brought down the courses, pregnant women had such bad blood and were subject to so many disorders that bleeding seemed essential. Sudell complained that 'It is too too common, especially amongst the Countrey-women, that if they be sick and be with child, they will not admit by no means to take Physick, or be let blood for fear of miscarriage'. Mauriceau on the other hand thought routine bleeding at four and seven months was so usual that most women, if they should neglect it, although they were otherwise well, would never believe they could be satisfactorily delivered, but he himself thought this was by no means always needful.[18]

Diet in the narrower sense of food and drink was subject to a host of rules and regulations. Always a tricky thing, in view of the need to keep the humoral balance right, it was even more difficult in pregnancy. Much of the advice about food was quite sensible, although it was of course based largely on the humoral properties of foods. Mauriceau counselled women to drink 'good old Wine, rather Claret than White, being well mixed with good running Fountain-Water, and not that which hath been long kept in Cisterns'. Ale and barley water were acceptable, but small drink not thought to be so good.

Orange juice taken with meals helped the digestion, broth mixed with egg yolk was nourishing and digestible, and after meals 'for the repressing of vapours fuming up into the head, alwaies stiptick and binding fruits are to be taken', such as pears, quinces and medlars. Culpeper thought it so important that pregnant women should eat well that he wished some State provision could be made to ensure such women should not go short of necessities, or what they might perhaps long for, and he thought their needs were worthy objects of rich neighbours' charity.

Forbidden foods included salads and spiced meats, and too much salt meat, which would make the child be born without nails, a sign of short life. Pregnant women were also to avoid lentils, beans, fried food and 'hot-seasoned Pyes and baked Meats, and especially Crust, because being hard of digestion, it extreamly overchargeth the stomach'. But Rueff also advised cutting out milk, fruit and cheese from the diet, and most authors thought milk and fish too phlegmatic to be wholesome. Towards the end of pregnancy oil and butter were thought to ease the labour. It was commonly believed toast was very strengthening, taken dipped in wine, or even applied externally. Furthermore a pregnant women was advised to eat toasted bread every day so that nothing would grow to the child.[19]

A particularly difficult problem arose when a pregnant woman longed for something unobtainable, or bad for her. It was well known that 'women with child haue oftentimes such disordinate appetite, by reason of some salt or sharp humor which is contained within the membranes of the stomacke, that they desire to eat Coles, Chalke, Ashes, Waxe, Salt-fish raw, yea and vnwatred; and to drink Veriuice, and Vineger, yea very dregs, so that it is impossible to hinder them'. In such a case they must have what they longed for, for fear they should fall into labour, or the child be born with the marks of some of the things they had so earnestly desired.[20]

Hare-lip was definitely caused either by fright at the starting of a hare, or by longing to eat hare. Therefore 'care is to be had, that speach bee not made of meate not to bee gotten before women conceived with childe'. One wonders what happened when the pregnant wives 'longed to bite off a piece of their Husbands Buttocks'.[21] Maubray thought a pregnant woman ought not to frequent gardens, where she might sit on some abortifacient herb, or see and covet some herb or fruit which might be bad for her if eaten, and equally bad if denied her.

We have already seen that the imagination was believed to act upon the foetus, therefore avoiding everything that might possibly mark the unborn child was an important part of the regimen. This included foods longed for, ugly sights and pictures, and any sudden fright. Maubray explained how these marks arose, and suggested a simple preventive remedy; 'if a *Mouse*, *Rat*, *Weazel*, *Cat*, or the like, leaps suddenly upon a *Woman* that has conceived, or if an *Apple*, *Pear*, *Plum*, *Cherry*, &c. fall upon any part of her *Body*; the MARK of the thing, (be what it will) is instantly *imprinted*, and will manifestly appear on the same *Part*, or *Member* of the CHILD: unless the *Woman* (in that very Moment) wipe *That Part* or *Member*, and move her *Hand* to some more remote, private, or convenient *Place* of the *Body*: which done, the MARK is actually averted, or at least stamped upon the *other Part* touch'd'.[22] According to Culpeper hare-lip could be avoided if the pregnant woman slit her smock at the sides like a shirt. It was also possible to take medicine against sudden frights, Sharp gives a prescription for one: '*Against sudden frights*. Take Mastick, Frankincense, of each one dram, Dragons blood, Myrtles, Bolearmoniak, Hermes berries, of each half a scruple, make them into powder and give half a dram at once with White Wine or Chicken broth'.

Women did blame these frights and sights for any peculiarity in their newborn children. A woman whose child was born face first and therefore much bruised told Mauriceau 'she always fear'd her Child would be so monstrous; because when she was young with Child of it, she fixed her looks very much upon a Blackmoor belonging to the Duke *de Guise*, who alwaies kept several of them'; Mauriceau did not ridicule her fears, but assured her the blackness was the result of the hard labour and would pass off.[23]

Maubray thought it unwise for pregnant women to play with pet animals for fear of marking the child, and one writer's objection to the practice of hanging felons in chains was mainly that pregnant women might be frighted by coming suddenly upon the sight, or perhaps miscarry because of the stench.[24]

There were other causes of deformed births believed in, less commonly. Rueff thought that a monster born at Cracow was to be attributed to God's will alone, 'yet not withstanding through the insight of our reason, we may perceive the detestable sinne of Sodomie in this Monster'. Bestial intercourse was, in the opinion of Dr Chamberlain, the most likely cause of a monstrous Tartar, captured by the Germans among the Turks, whose picture depicting a head and neck like a horse had lately been on show, 'those beastly and unnaturall commixtures being familiar and usuall amongst those bruitish Infidells'.[25]

Fortunately, although 'it cannot be denied, but that Devils transforming themselves into human Shapes, may abuse both Men and Women, and with wicked People use Copulation', no children could be engendered.[26] Other horrid consequences might ensue however, as in this case: 'a certaine Harlot, having her body lasciviously abused of the Divell, in the night, comming in the shape of a man, did streight way fall into a most great sicknesse, so that her wombe and privity were quickly consumed with a consumption or rotting *Gangræna*, so that . . . her intralls also and parts about her secret members did fall out of her body'.[27]

The real-life case of Mary Tofts, who in 1726 pretended to have given birth to a litter of rabbits, and convinced both the local man-midwife and the anatomist to the King before her trick was finally exposed, shows how uncritically the most extraordinary stories about pregnancy and childbirth could be received, and not only among the uneducated.[28]

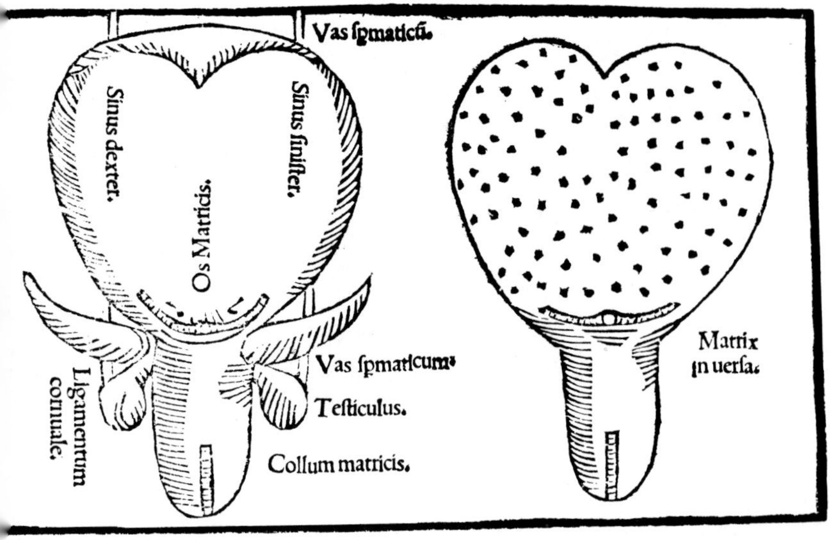


Plate 1. The uterus and ovaries, and the uterus shown internally (B. da Carpi: *Isagoge breves* 1522 f. 52r). By courtesy of the Wellcome Trustees.

Plate 2. The uterus and reproductive organs, after Vesalius. Fig. II shows the imaginary bypass vessels, fig. IV the semi-compartmented uterus in cross-section (T. Johnson, tr: *The works....of Ambrose Parey* 1634 p. 127). By courtesy of the Wellcome Trustees.

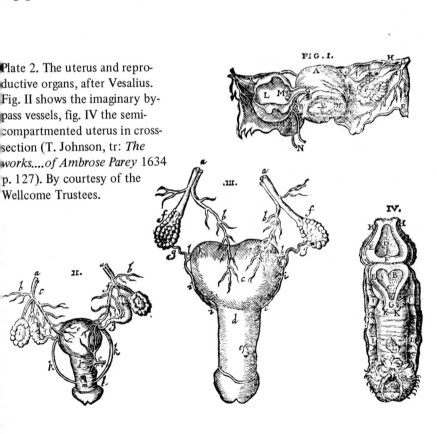

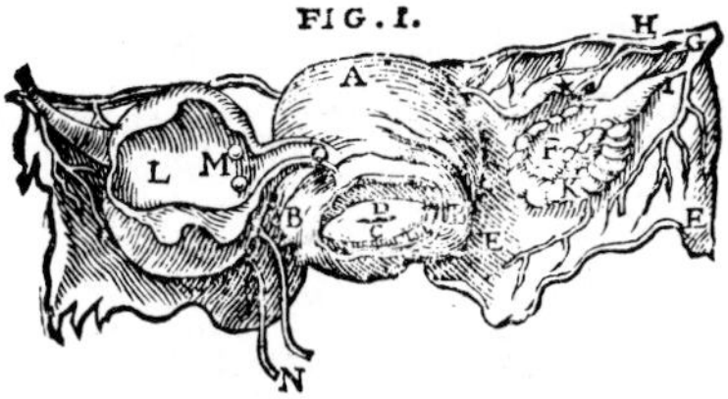


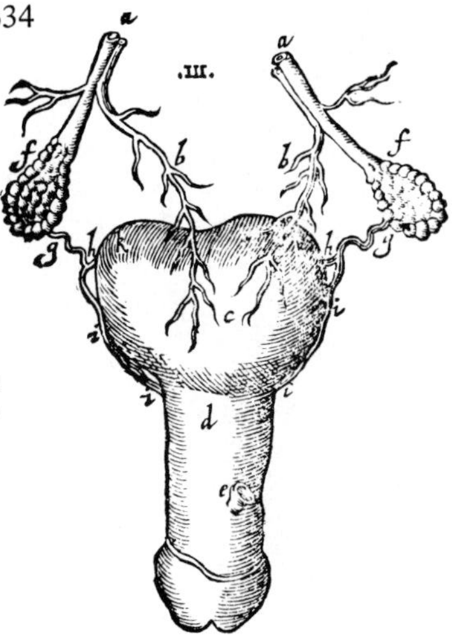


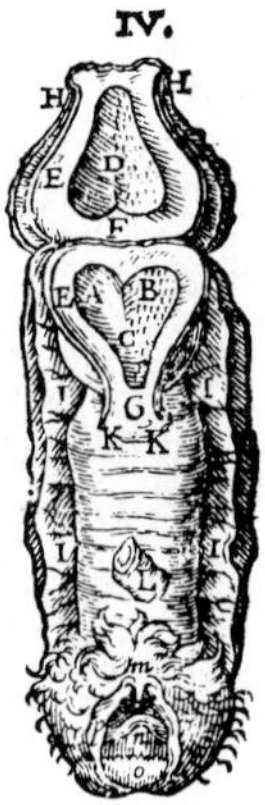


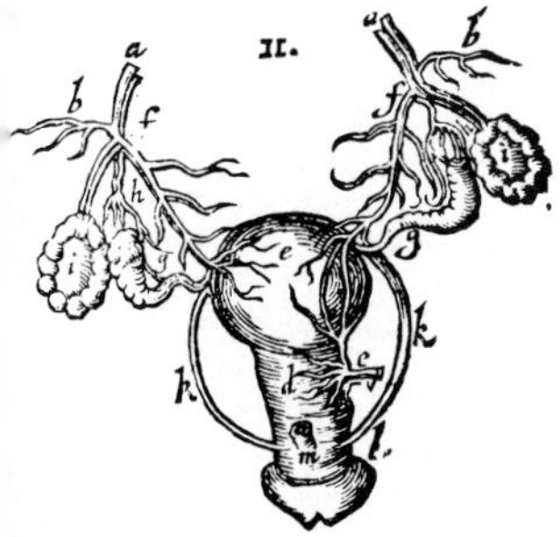

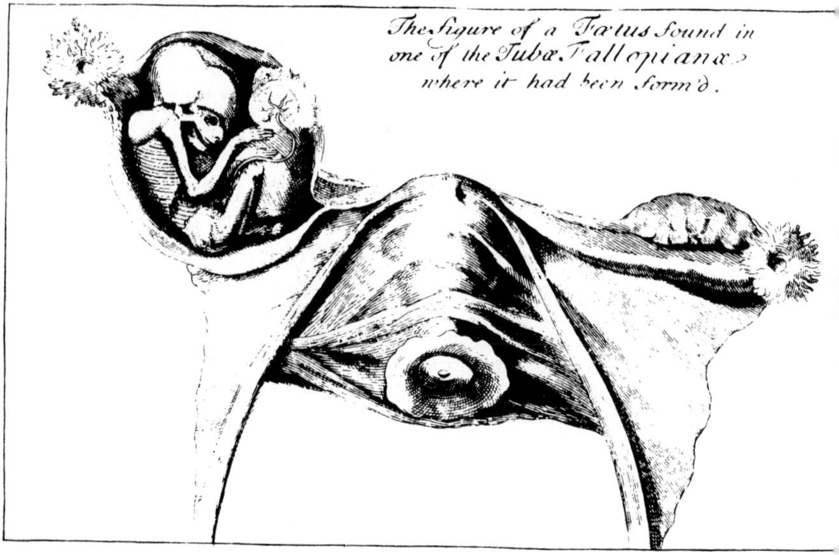

The figure of a Fœtus found in
one of the Tubæ Fallopianæ
where it had been form'd.


Plate 3 (*above*). A very early representation of ectopic gestation. (P. Dionis: *A general treatise of midwifery* 1719 facing p. 82). By courtesy of the Wellcome Trustees.

Plate 4 (*below* and *above right*). Three stages in the formation of the foetus. Note in the third figure (c) the band representing the placenta, and the foetal position (J. Rueff: *The expert midwife* 1637). By courtesy of the Wellcome Trustees.

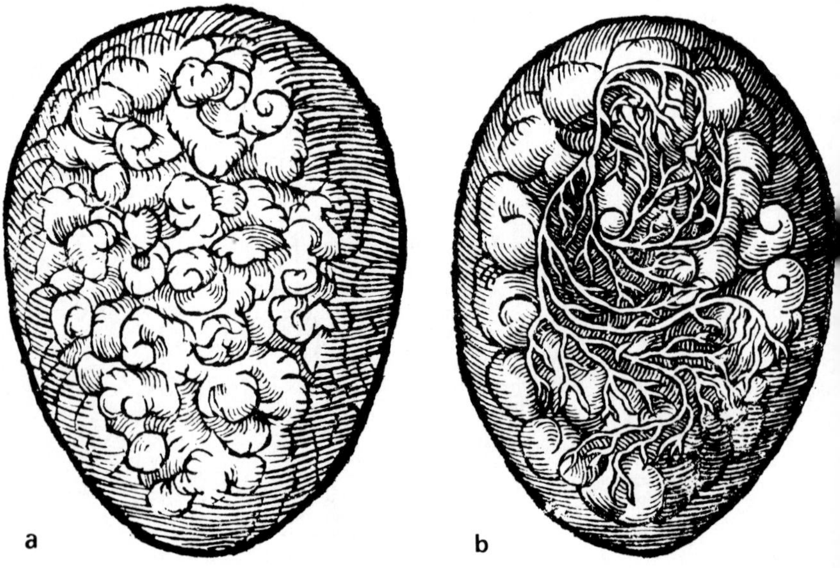

c

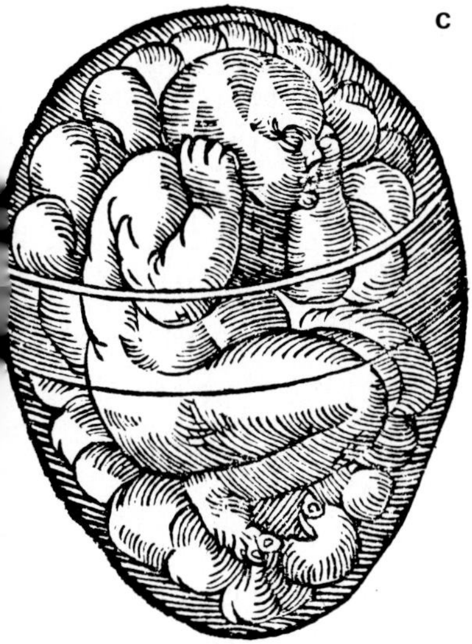

Plate 5 (*below*). The foetus at eighteen days gestation (J. Wolveridge: *Speculum matricis* 1671 facing p. 12). By courtesy of the Wellcome Trustees.

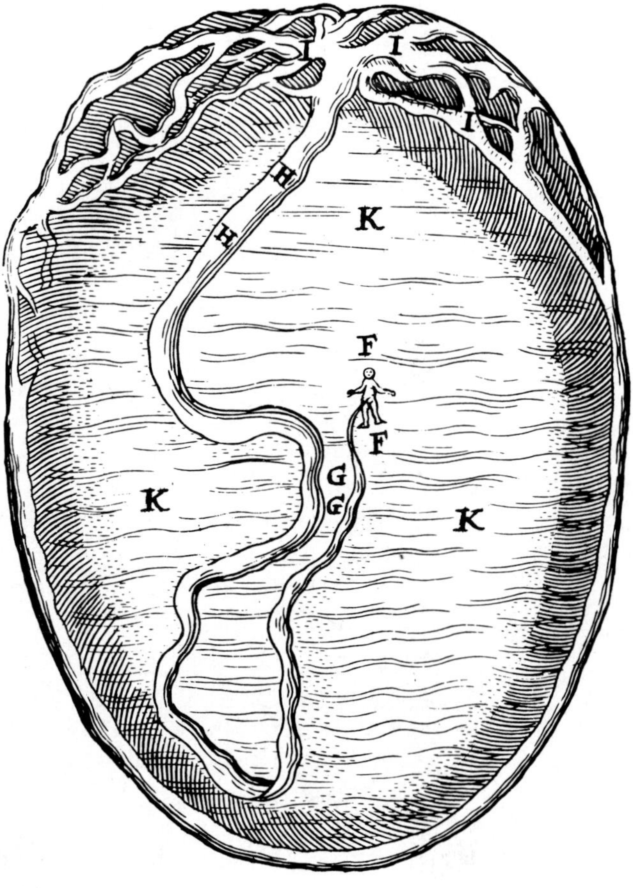

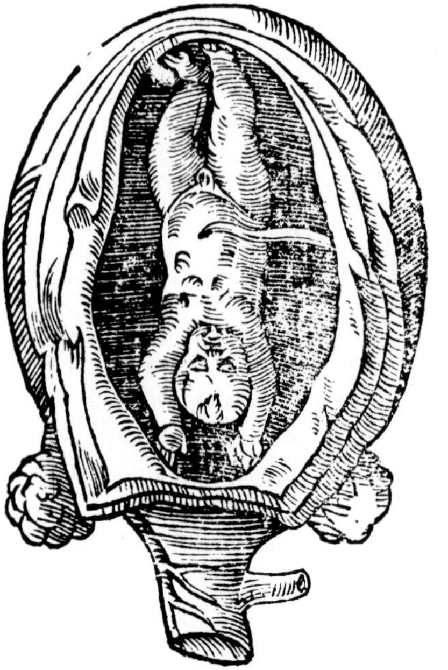

Plate 6 (*left*). A possible mal-presentation (J. Rueff: *The expert midwife* 1637 p. 123). By courtesy of the Wellcome Trustees.

Plate 7 (*below*). A surgeon reducing a prolapse (*Die Handschrift des Schnitt und Augenarztes Caspar Stromayr.... 1559* Berlin, Idra 1925 p. 332). By courtesy of the Wellcome Trustees.

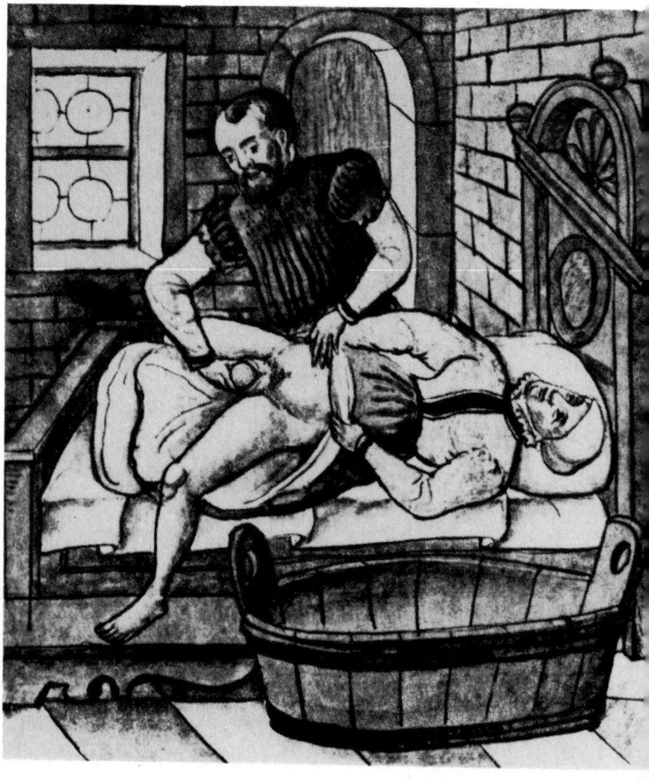

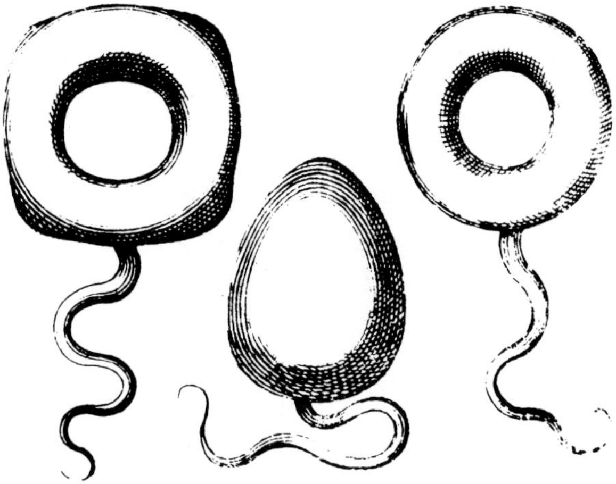

Plate 8 (*above*). Pessaries for the support of prolapse (F. Mauriceau: *The diseases of women with child, and in child-bed* 1697 facing p. 128). By courtesy of the Wellcome Trustees.

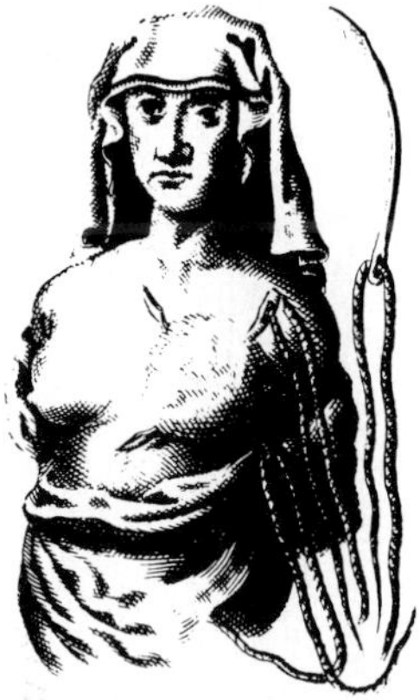

Plate 9 (*right* and *below*). Mastectomy (J. Scultetus: *Armamentarium chirurgicum* 1656-7 p. 146). By courtesy of the Wellcome Trustees.

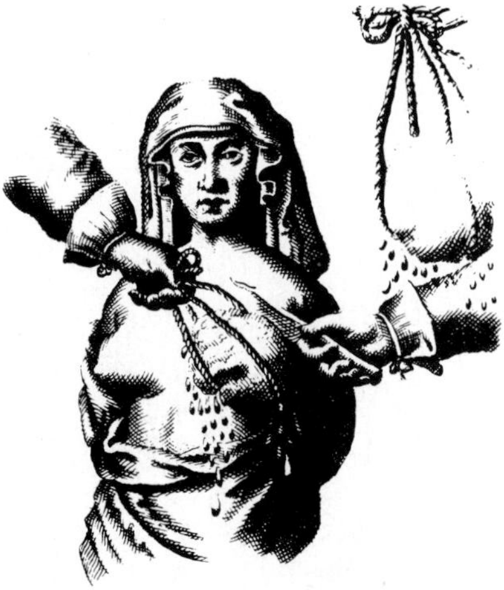

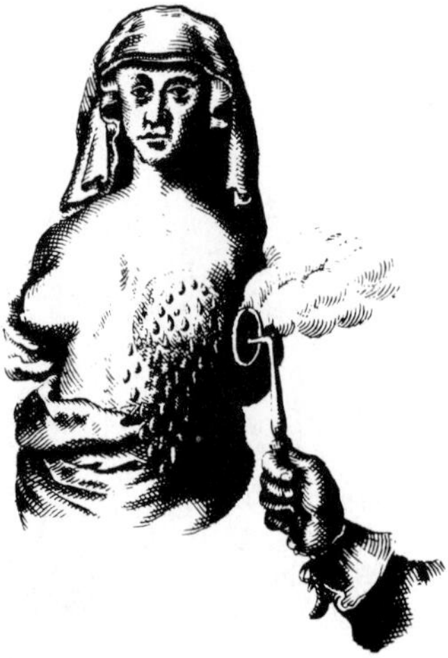

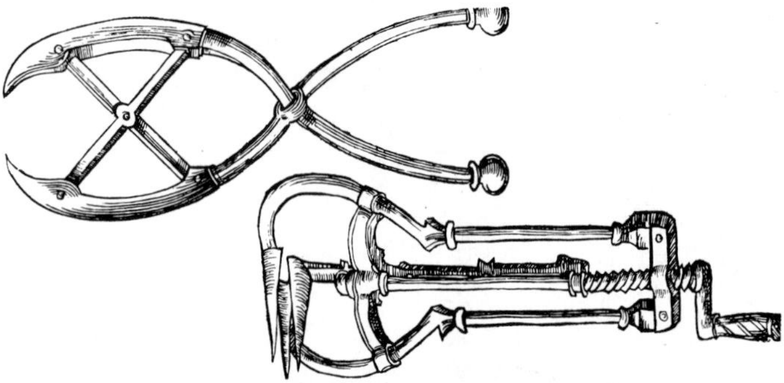

Plate 10a (*above*). Obstetrical instruments (J. Rueff: *The expert midwife* 1637 p. 105). By courtesy of the Wellcome Trustees. Plate 10b (*below*). Obstetrical instruments (F. Mauriceau: *The diseases of women with child, and in child-bed* 1697 facing p. 128). By courtesy of the Wellcome Trustees.

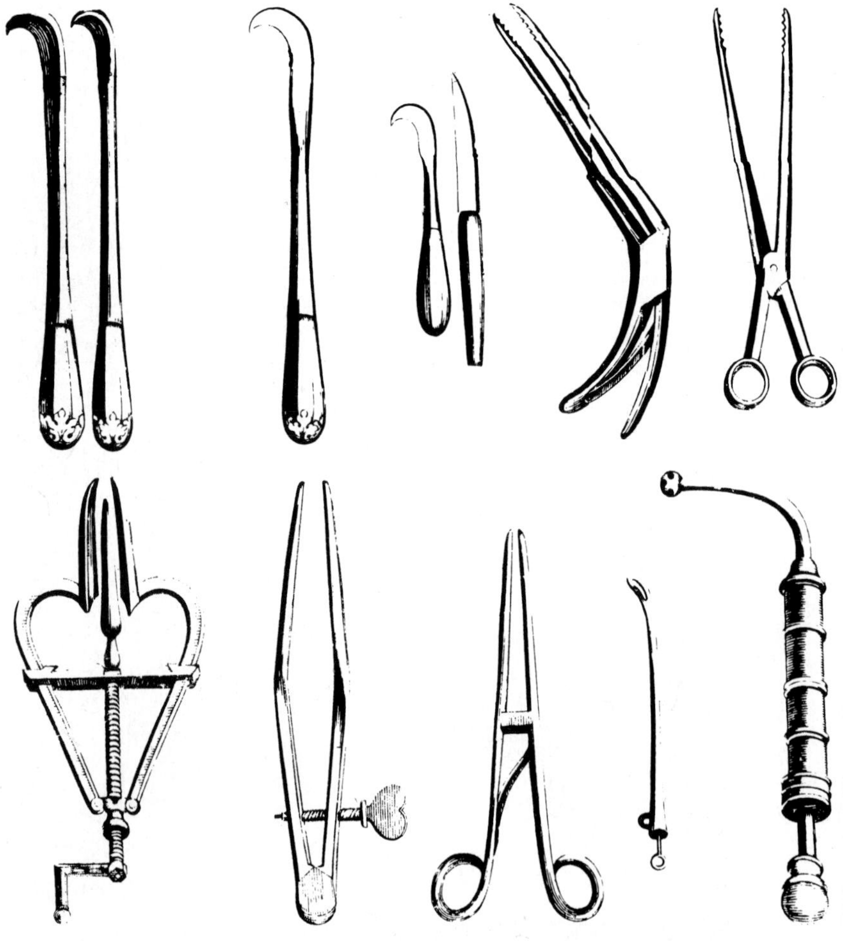

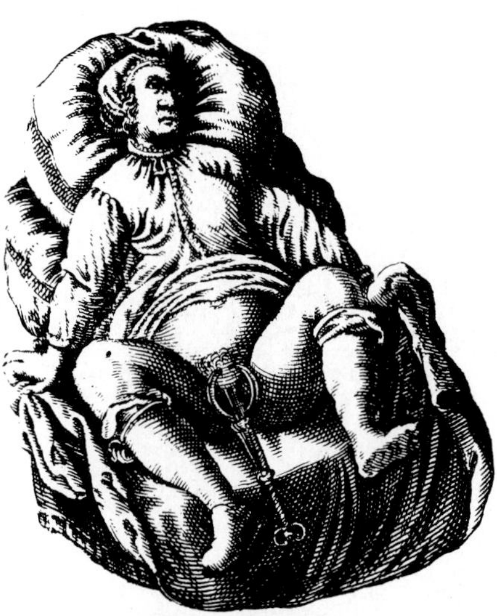

Plate 11 (*left*). The vaginal speculum in use (J. Scultetus: *Armamentarium chirurgicum* 1656-7 p. 164). By courtesy of the Wellcome Trustees.

Plate 12 (*below*). Caesarean section; extraction of the foetus (S. Mercurio: *La commare o riccoglitrice* 1601 p. 217). By courtesy of the Wellcome Trustees.

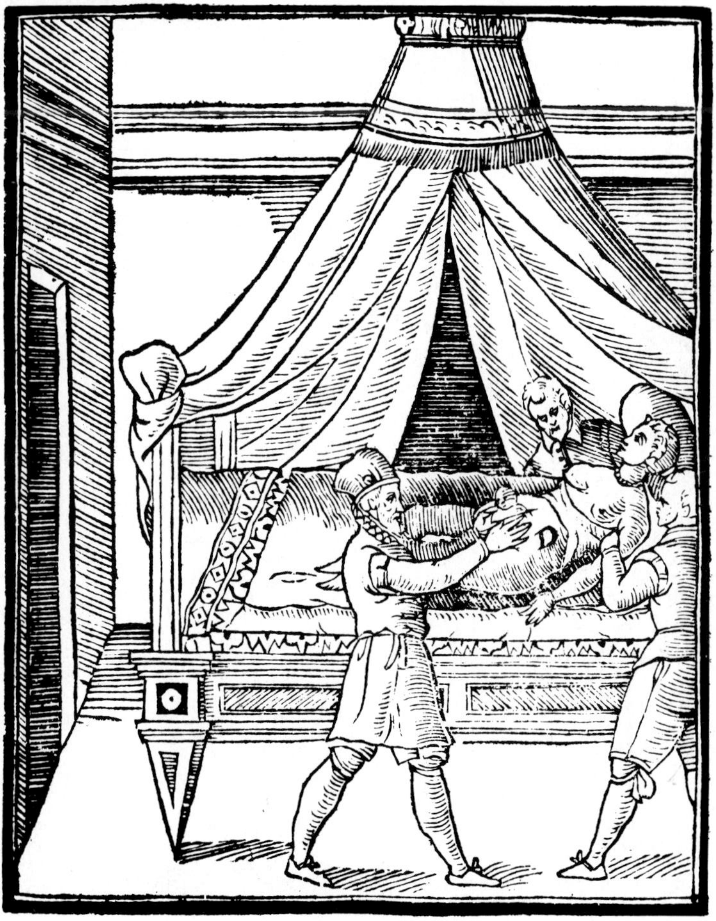

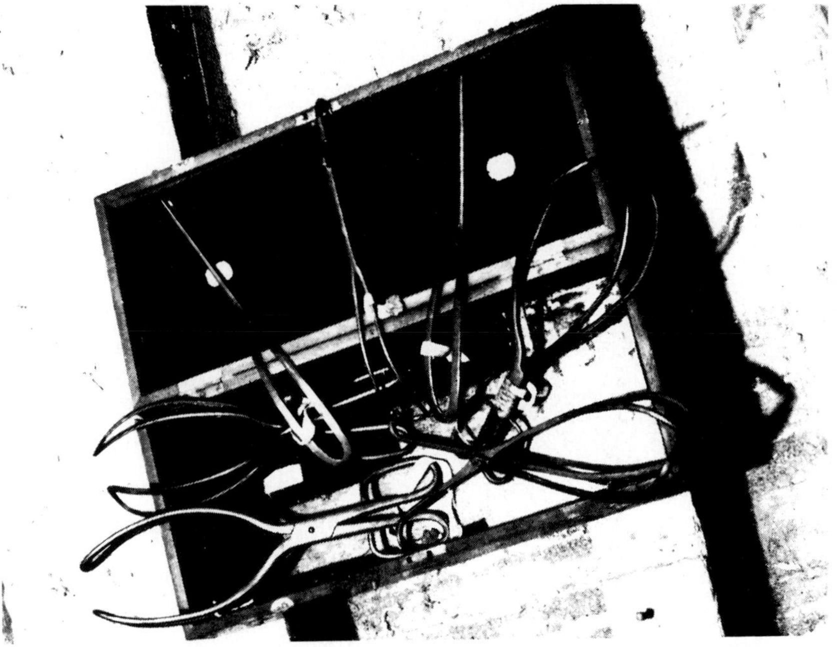

Plate 13a (*above*). The forceps found at Woodham Hall, Essex, once the home of the Chamberlen family. By kind permission of R. C. Percival FRCOG. Plate 13b (*below*). The forceps as used by Giffard, and Freke's model incorporating handles which doubled as crochets (W. Giffard: *Cases in midwifry* 1734 Plate I). By courtesy of the Wellcome Trustees.

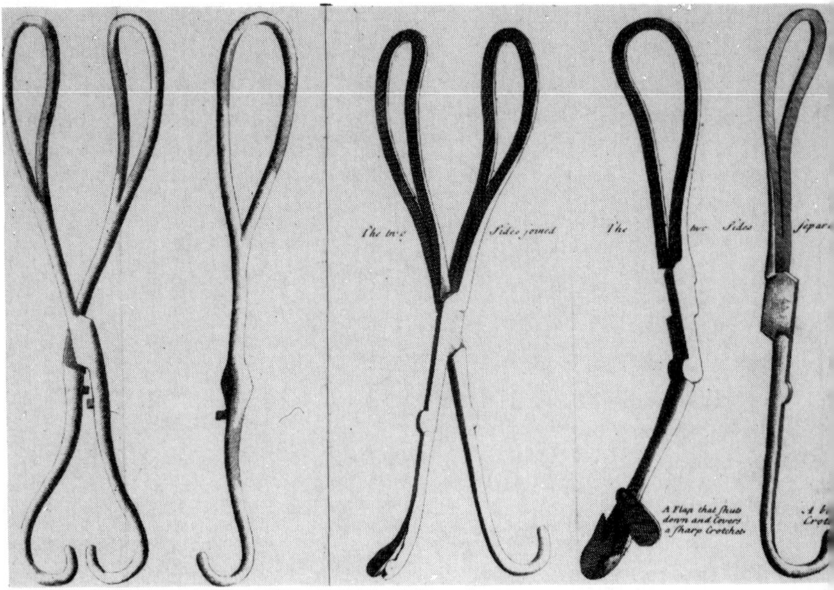

*Chapter Eight*

# Pregnancy Prevention and Promotion

Trotula quoted Galen's opinion that women with narrow vulvas and tight wombs ought not to have husbands lest they died if they conceived; she continued 'But since they cannot all abstain they need our help . . . remove the testicles from a weasel and let it be left alive. Let the woman carry those testicles with her on her bosom . . . and she will not conceive'. But by the time our authors wrote, the attitude of the church had so hardened against contraception and abortion that any such frank statement would have been impossible.

It has been pointed out that mediaeval authors furnished contraceptive advice under the specious guise of advice against sterility: 'The kinds of 'extrinsic' causes mentioned by these authors are so clearly the result of deliberate human choice that the recital of them cannot be for diagnostic purposes only. John [of Gaddesden] is not aiming to help a doctor whose patient is mysteriously sterile because she has blundered by wearing the heart of a mule; Magnino is not visualizing a patient who has inadvertently used a cabbage-seed pessary or hung saxifrage over her bed. The information is given not to cure sterility, but to indicate how contraception is accomplished'.[1]

Without much stretching of the probabilities however, it is hard to read any such humane, if devious, intentions into the medical writings of the sixteenth and seventeenth centuries. This is admittedly a subjective view, since contraceptive information is quite readily obtainable from them, but the authors themselves are so unanimous in their condemnation of all such practices, of which they do not pretend to be ignorant, that one must either accuse them of the rankest hypocrisy, or accept that any contraceptive use of their information was not their intention.

It is clear however that on certain social levels both contraception and abortion were familiar. There seems to have been a sub-culture, largely female, where such ideas were exchanged and where the attempts of women to control their own fertility were active.[2] Towards the end of the time indeed the notion that it was possibly not whores and the mothers of bastards alone who might have an interest in avoiding pregnancy did begin to surface, albeit cautiously. Nevertheless the whole tone of the midwiferies assumed that every woman wanted children, and only the most depraved would dream of avoiding this obligation of marriage. As Sharp put it: 'To conceive with child is the earnest desire if not of all yet of most women'.

It could not be denied that much of the information intended to prevent sterility and miscarriage could by a simple process of inversion be made to serve precisely the opposite purpose. Apart from the offence to female modesty which worried many of these authors, they also worried about the possible perversion of their advice. Raynald referred to the objection that 'summe wyckydly disposyd person shold abuse such medicynes as be here declaryd for a goud pourpose, to sume dyuellysshe and lewd vse. What I meane by the lewde vse of them, they that haue vnderstandynge, ryght soone wyll perceaue'.[3] He could do no more than disclaim any such intention and point out that the same could be said of holy writ itself, and many other good and necessary things.

Authors did include some warnings which sound peculiar, but they seem rather anxious to be compendious and uncritical of their sources than actuated by any ulterior motive. Rueff, for instance, noted among external causes of abortion 'if a woman conceived with childe, doe tread upon a serpent, viper, the egge of a Crow (as some doe write) or a dead serpent with two heads named Amphisbæna'; but he could not surely have intended his pregnant female readers to go out looking for vipers and crow's eggs to tread on and thus procure abortion.[4] There are of course many examples of less esoteric advice which could perfectly well have been turned to contraceptive use in practice, but there is no evidence that that was the author's intention.

Later authors did seem more aware that unbridled fecundity was not desired by every woman. Mauriceau remarked that the opening of the cervix in copulation was 'purely natural, and not voluntary; which is not amiss: for if the motion of this Orifice depend on the Will of the Women, there would be many who would thereby hinder Conception in the use of Copulation; and there would be many wicked enough to expel and reject, at pleasure, the Seed which they have conceived'.[5] *Aristotle's experienced midwife* made the same point: 'for were it otherway, there would not be so many Bastards begotten as there are; nor would many married Women have so many Children, were it at their own Choice'.

Medical authors did not suggest contraceptive measures even for therapeutic reasons. Pechey, among others, pointed out that when a birth injury to the perineum has once occurred 'it is very difficult to prevent the like in the following Travail . . . wherefore it were to be wished for greater security against the like accidents, that the Woman should have no more Children';[7] he did not, however, offer any suggestion how this might be achieved. Similarly Willughby, though clearly much distressed by the gloomy prognosis in childbirth for his rachitic patients, never once suggested any means by which they could avert their own probable death.

However, it was conceded by many authors that women might themselves seek abortion or attempt contraception, however morally objectionable such action might be. Many of the warnings about the difficulty of diagnosing pregnancy were intended to prevent the involvement of some unwary practitioner in such a scheme.

Riverius advised that when a patient complained of stopped courses it behoved the doctor to take note of all the physical signs 'lest the Physitian be deceived by Women that would dissemble their being with Child, and lest he should rashly prescribe Medicines to provoke terms to Women with Child'.[8] Sadler thought one of the objections to uroscopy was that, since the doctor could not diagnose pregnancy from the urine, he might prescribe some strong cathartic or diuretic to a pregnant woman and so cause abortion.[9]

Willughby knew of a gentlewoman who persuaded a friend of his, a doctor of medicine and a man-midwife, to extract a false conception, which turned out to be a child: 'At the sight thereof hee was much troubled (hee told it to mee with a great deale of sorrow) and said unto her, that hee was displeased with her evil doings'. She nevertheless afterwards persuaded other physicians, knowing nothing of her former dealings, to abort her on other occasions, and eventually died 'By physick'.[10]

Dr John Casaubon recorded in his diary his misgivings about one Mary Best who had strange fits: 'let blood in ye foot by my Directions, I pray God she were not whorish and did it thincking to avoyd being w$^{th}$ Child'.[11] Portal and another doctor declined to bleed a patient in the foot, suspecting she was pregnant, although the midwife thought not, but she aborted in any case of a macerated foetus.

The advice of the famous French midwife Louise Bourgeois to her daughter included warnings not to give abortifacients, and this was also a clause in the seventeenth-century midwife's oath.

But abortionists did exist. According to Brugis they were mostly empirics and illiterate unqualified practitioners, 'and these kinde of creatures will give a dram . . . make an abort if need be, keep downe their paps, hinder conception, procure lust, make them able with provocatives, and now and then step in themselves'.[12] Rueff said that there were old witches and harlots who were applied to by women whose first attempts at abortion by tight lacing had failed, who would send them to the apothecaries for medicines, and if these did not work, told them to open a vein in the foot, which finally brought about the abortion. In other cases women who had successfully brought on an abortion told each other how it was done: 'Besides, also many Midwives, and also Chirurgions, and unskilfull Physicians, sometimes over-credulous, doe counsell & advise such things to great evil and mischiefe'.[13]

Lists of medicines to bring on the terms included such items as rue and savin, which were still popular abortifacients for self-administration in the nineteenth century, and according to Raynald few or no women were ignorant of such things. De la Motte by way of warning reported that 'a young woman, out of her wits at being big with child, used all she could think of to get rid of it, as decoctions of *Rue*, *Savin*, and other herbs of this nature, with frequent *Bleeding* in the arm and foot', which caused her death, but not the abortion.[14]

Among individual, real-life, examples savin was used in an Elizabethan incest case, and at Holt in Derby in 1667.[15] Women were presented in the church courts in the sixteenth and seventeenth centuries for administering love potions which were really abortifacients.[16] An eighteenth-century husband who had got his wife's sister with child obtained some abortifacient pills from a midwife in Fleet Street for the sister to take, but they did not work.[17] The trial of Eleanor Merriman for abortion using iron instruments was reported in the *Gentleman's Magazine* in August 1732; she was found guilty and sentenced to the pillory and three years imprisonment. According to Bartholin the cervix after conception was too tightly closed for whores who tried to draw out a conception to succeed, but it seems quite likely that this method was in successful use.[18]

Contraception, as opposed to abortion, seems to have been largely confined to charms and amulets, and to such methods as the church considered marital sins; namely coitus interruptus, intercourse in any position other than the approved 'missionary' position, anal and oral intercourse. Culpeper referring to Onan's sin drily observed 'for this God slew him: I beleeve God hath been more merciful to many in *England* in the same case'.[19] Sharp made a veiled reference to men and women who mutilated themselves on purpose, or used destructive means to cause barrenness, which she thought unjustifiable. Barrough might possibly have been dropping a hint however when he warned those who desired children to avoid eating rue, for 'rewe doth altogether corrupt & destroy seede'.[20]

Although the condom and the contraceptive sponge both existed in the seventeenth century there is not the faintest suggestion that any of the medical writers even knew of them.[21] Not even the use of the condom against venereal disease is hinted at, though the disease itself is discussed. Even more surprisingly, though breast feeding was beginning to be actively encouraged for all classes, Dionis alone mentioned lactation as a contraceptive: 'Married Women have ordinarily a Child every Year; but those who give suck *one* in two or three *only*: which ought to induce Mothers to suckle their own Children, because Women with Child are subject to a great many more Diseases than Nurses'.[22] Women themselves of course were probably quite well aware of this, though wealthy women were either less so, or preferred repeated pregnancy to lactation.[23]

The promotion of fertility received much attention, and the daily rules and regulations for pregnant women had as their chief object the prevention of miscarriage. Articles of diet to increase seed, promote heat and provoke lust included the flesh of small birds, especially sparrows, on the principle that 'All Creatures that are fruitful, being eaten, make those fruitful that eat them'. Other such foods included eggs, milk, rice boiled in milk, beans, peas, onions, garlic, leeks, French beans, radishes, hazel and almond nuts, marzipan, cinnamon, cardamom, cloves, ginger and saffron.

If dietary methods and the right conduct of intercourse alone did not produce the desired conception there were other methods which could be tried. If the barrenness was due to humoral causes the usual ways of purging, bleeding and altering the humours were obviously the first thing to try. The well known pills grana angelica, one dram taken every 14 days, were recommended. On the other hand Spanish fly taken to excess could cause priapism: 'It is not to be imagined what pains some have undergone, who by indiscreet taking of *Cantharides* have fallen into this grievous distemper'.[24] Topical applications to the penis were no doubt safer; oil of mastich and wormwood with a few grains of musk and civet would help erection. Or the woman could take in wine the dried and powdered navel-string of a first-born boy that had never touched the ground; powder of bull's pizzle, or powder of fox's testicles, one dram taken in sheep's milk, also helped barrenness. Also,

'Several highly commend the Chimical Oil of the lesser sweet Marjoram, mixt with the Runnet of a Hare, and some few grains of musk to facilitate Conception.'[25]

There were also amulets reputed to cause mutual love and fruitfulness; the heart of a male quail carried about the man, and the heart of a female quail carried about the woman for example. A loadstone worn about the neck had the same effect, as did the eagle stone. These stones were also useful to prevent miscarriage once conception had occurred. If all else failed a visit to the mineral baths might cure barrenness: 'very many women in this Condition, do flock unto such Baths, as to a Sanctuary'.[26]

Paré declined to suggest any remedy where the sterility was caused by 'inchantment, magick, witching, and enchanted knots, bands and ligatures, for those causes belong not to physick, neither may they bee taken away by the remedies of our art'. Riverius thought it helped to forsake their houses, beds, clothes, and other household stuff, where the charms might often be concealed. He also claimed the pizzle of a wolf worn about the woman would counteract such spells. If a man was impotent because of witchcraft he could try taking a draught of cold water that dropped from the mouth of a young stallion while drinking, saved in a little vessel.

Culpeper observed that charms could be worn to forestall impotence caused by witchcraft; 'But suppose the mischief be already done, and the man cannot give his W[i]fe due benevolence, how may it be helped? In this I will tell you no more than I have known tried, the cure is easie, and was done by the Man only making water through his Wives Wedding-Ring'.[27]

Once conception was achieved however there were numerous means to avert miscarriage, from amulets to medicines. 'If signs of abortion appear, the usual way is, to lay a Tost, sopt in Muskadel to her Navel, and many times it doth good' according to Culpeper, but syrup of garden tansy he thought had a magnetic virtue which made it even more useful, and he advised midwives always to have some handy, though it was not in the official *Dispensatory* of the Royal College of Physicians.[28]

Women took plantain seed the whole time of pregnancy to prevent abortion, and this was thought sound practice by writers. Fluxes of any sort which might cause abortion could be cured by 15 or 30 drops of liquid laudanum in a glass of canary at bedtime. 'Tea infused in Ale, like Sage-Ale, and a Draught drank every Morning, is most excellent for such Women as are subject to Miscarriages.'[29] Women also had great faith in crimson silk shredded up and taken in the yolk of an egg to ward off abortion after a fall or injury. Mauriceau considered this remedy superstitious and ridiculous, but 'one may give it to those that desire it to content them, because these Remedies, though useless, can yet do no hurt'.[30]

In the case of most of the measures mentioned in this chapter probably that is the best that could be said of them.

*Chapter Nine*

# Gynaecology

Diseases of the female reproductive organs were from ancient times believed to be both very common and very serious; Harvey wrote: 'No man, (who is but never so litle versed in such matters) is ignorant, what grievous *Symptomes*, the Rising, Bearing down, and Perversion, and Convulsion of the *Womb* do excite; what horrid extravagancies of minde, what Phrensies, Melancholy Distempers, and Outragiousness, the *præternatural Diseases* of the Womb do induce, as if the affected Persons were inchanted: as also how many difficult *Diseases*, the depraved effluxion of the Terms, or the use of *Venus* much intermitted, and long desired do foment'.[1]

Because menstruation was regarded as essential to health in women of mature age, as well as essential to conception, menstrual disorders received considerable attention in the textbooks. Amenorrhoea was regarded as the most serious condition, and included not only secondary and primary amenorrhoea 'if the Terms be stopped . . . Or if they never did appear', but also scanty menses, 'when women are not sufficiently or conveniently purged, at their monthly seasons'. Freind said that 'a *diminution of the Menses* is by far the most frequent Distemper, and almost *epidemick* among *Virgins* . . . there is hardly found any Disease in *Girls*, which has not this either for its Cause, or Attendant'.[2]

This malady was potentially very dangerous however; according to Riverius 'the stoppage of the Terms is very dangerous, and many great diseases come thereof, and some in the Womb it self, as swellings, imposthumes, and Ulcers; others in the whol Body, and divers parts thereof, as Feavers, Obstructions, evil Habits, Loathing, Dropsie, Heart-ach, Cough, short Breathing, Fainting, sore Eyes, Madness, Melancholly, Headach, Joynt-gout, and the like'.[3]

The chief reason why young women did not begin to menstruate was of course humoral, because their complexion was too hot and dry, so that they consumed their nourishment as completely as men, and nothing was left to be evacuated. Culpeper thought the errors of physicians were sometimes to blame, when they wrongly prescribed blood-letting in the arm to virgins who were 'out of frame' at puberty, and thus dried up and diverted the blood which ought to begin to break out by the womb.

This could have very far reaching consequences such as depression and hot flushes in middle age: 'elderly women, whose courses were stopt when they were young, are troubled oftentimes with the Spleen, & hypochondriack Melancholy . . . when the thin part of the blood is inflamed they grow very hot, and red in the Face, but that lasts not long'.[4]

Even after the courses began to come regularly and normally, it needed very little disturbance to stop them. Going into cold water, for example, at the time of the menses, or overheating the lower parts and drying up the blood by carrying coals under one's coat in the winter time, or even drinking too much tea.

Bearing in mind the horrid consequences which might follow stoppage of the courses it was hardly surprising that such a stoppage complicating another disease presented the physician with a knotty problem. Copious blood-letting in the foot was clearly needed for the amenorrhoea, but what should be done if the complicating disease required some other, perhaps quite opposite treatment? Pechey came to the conclusion that 'in slight Diseases, and in such as will bear a Truce, experience has taught me that it is best to bleed in the Foot; for the indication from the Courses stopt is more to be minded than a small Disease, and therefore they ought to be provoked, first by Ligatures, Cupping-glasses, Frictions, and Medicines, and afterwards you must provide for the Disease: But if the Disease be violent, as a Quinsie, Pleurisie, or the like; then certainly those Remedies must be given which the Disease requires, without consideration of the Veins of the Foot'.[5]

Besides the measures mentioned by Pechey for stoppage of the courses, issues in the legs were advised, also brimstone or bitumen baths, leeches applied to the haemorrhoid veins, vomits (but only those that 'may worke both wayes, lest working onely upward, it should too much turne backe the humour'), and medicines such as hiera picra or '*Pil. Arabica* which the Apothecary will help you to, two scruples, and of Oil of Amber four drops mixed with it; be in your Chamber that day, and drinking Posset, as is ordinary in taking Physick'.[6] Sweating, preferably in a hothouse, was also good. Grown women could use medicated pessaries, but fumigations were better for virgins.[7]

Riverius clearly regretted the good old days when he quoted a case where Galen cured a woman that had her courses stopped eight months, by bleeding a pint and a half the first day, the next one pint, the third not above half a pint, or eight ounces. From which Riverius concluded it was perfectly acceptable to let women blood copiously in such cases 'although the women of our Age will not endure it'.

The treatment of excessive courses was similar but opposite — the bleeding, 'as much as her strength can bear', issues, cupping and so forth were to be applied to the upper parts of the body to make revulsion of the blood. There were also medicines appropriate to the condition, such as plasters to the navel, either the plaster against ruptures, or the hysterical plaster, or Vigo's plaster for fractures, 'which is most excellent; and works it's effect without heating the Part'. Smoke of burnt frogs as a fumigation could be used, and rather more agreeably, allum baths and a potion of orange peel water.[8]

Some of these remedies were also applied in dysmenorrhoea, though far less attention was paid to this than to stoppage of the courses. Either painful menstruation was relatively rare, or seldom brought to the attention of medical men. Pechey pointed out that 'It is a Disease more incident to Maids than married Women, because the Veins of the Womb are less open in them, than in those who brought forth Children. It happens sometimes from a corruption of the blood, that is, from the drossiness and thickness thereof, and then the blood clots together; and there is a great pain long before the Flowers begin to come down'.[9] The usual cupping, bleeding, leeching and so on was supplemented in this case by doses of Venice treacle and mithridate, and by opium as a last resort.

Sadler pointed out that in some cases of suppressed courses 'the Cotyledones are so closed up, that nothing but copulation will open them', a characteristic which links this condition with a group of diseases including hysteria and chlorosis, in which unsatisfied desire, and therefore unevacuated seed, was at least a contributory factor. Hysteria in the modern sense was undoubtedly one of the problems included in 'fits of the mother', but it seems evident that a large number of otherwise unexplained symptoms were, if they occurred in a female, simply taken to be 'fits of the mother'. Hysteria in this wide seventeenth-century sense was 'common and very troublesom'.

In the fifteenth century 'suffocation of the mother' was caused by the womb literally rising out of its place and compressing the heart and lungs so that the sufferer fell down breathless in a swoon. The cause was the natural coldness of the uterus (all membranes were cold) which, if excessive, caused it to seek heat from parts of the body such as the heart and liver which were naturally hot. A hard swelling could be felt about the navel during these fits, and a choking sensation in the throat. The swoons were sometimes so profound and lasted so long the victim might be taken for dead.

Even at this early date it was suggested that corrupt menstrual blood or seed were causative factors,[10] and when the anatomical discoveries of the sixteenth century demonstrated that the womb was tied so fast with four ligaments that it was impossible for it to move to the upper parts, this notion was developed into a more modern explanation. Culpeper rather dismissively announced, 'my opinion is, that the disease you call the fits of the Mother, is nothing but a windiness of the Womb'.

Barrough thought the womb was stretched by retained menses or seed. According to Sharp, 'it is most commonly the widowes disease, who were wont to use Copulation, and are now constrained to live without it; when the seed is thus retained it corrupts, and sends up filthy vapours to the brain'. Sudell thought that it would help devise methods of cure if the route by which the vapours ascended were known, but according to another author 'the vapours . . . rise from the putrified blood to the head, through the Arteries that run along through the neck, passing by both parts of the infundibulum into the fore-part of the head'.[11]

Supporting evidence for the vapours theory was drawn from misinterpreted autopsy findings. Women's stones were full of wheyish seed 'when Women are in good health, but when they are sickly they seem like bladders full of a clear watry humour, and sometimes of a yellow colour like Saffron, and will stink, so that it oftentimes causeth the strangling of the Mother, which Midwives call fits of the Mother'.[12] A certain noble young damsel was found after death to have 'one stone . . . swelled to the greatness of a large hand-bal, being filled with a saffron-color'd humor, very stinking, and sending forth a filthy and poysonsom kind of vapor'. Thus is was now clear that the lump formerly believed to be the uterus rising up 'was not the Womb, but the Stones, with that blind Vessel, which from *Fallopius* the finder or first Observer thereof is called Fallopious his Trumpet'.[13] Sharp said these structures 'when they are full swoln with vapours and corrupt seed, they stir to and fro, and come up to the navel'.

Furthermore, the reason why men did not suffer from the disease was not so much that they had no uterus, but the different quality of men's seed. Maubray thought it was because men, by nocturnal pollutions or other ways, always eliminated their seed from the body, whereas women's remained within 'and consequently by a long *Detention* there, may be converted into VENOM, or a *Poysonous Humour*'.[14]

By the time Maubray wrote this however, the vapours theory in its turn was out of fashion, and the idea that women had no seed necessitated a yet newer explanation to be found. Some bold spirits even began to suggest that men might suffer from the disease.[15] The problem was now taken to be convulsions of the nerves: 'these plexus of Nerves are chiefly affected in Hysterick Fits, and are Convulsive, and often happen when the Womb is not at all in fault; and the Ball that seems to rise from the bottom of the Belly in these Fits, and to beat strongly about the Navel, which is usually supposed to be the rising of the Womb, is nothing but a Convulsion of these Nerves; for some Men are troubled with the same Symptom.'[16] Or in Willis's terms, 'what is vulgarly said to be done by Vapours . . . is nothing else, but the parts of the Membranes and Nervous ductus's forc'd successively into Contractions'.[17]

Pechey held that 'this whole Disease is occasioned by the Animal Spirits being not rightly disposed, and not by seed and menstruous blood corrupted, and sending up malignant Vapours . . . the fomes of the Disease does not lurk in matter . . . yet it must be confessed that the confusion of the Spirits produces putrid humors in the Body'. These disordered spirits were responsible for the emotional lability of hysterical women: 'Nor is it to be doubted, that weeping and laughing fits, which often seise hysterical women without any occasion, are procured by the Animal Spirits forcing themselves violently upon the Organs that perform these Animal functions'.[18]

Dr Chamberlain considered the mental symptoms 'their *frenzies*, or *frantick fits*, their *dumb silence*, and indeed inability to speak or utter themselves, their strange *fancies* of fear, some times loathing their lives, yet fearing beyond measure to *die*', resulted from 'sympathy' between the womb and the brain.[19] As early as the sixteenth century Barrough observed that 'it causeth sorrow & sadness, & dejection of the minde', and thought 'yong folke, and such as be prone to leacherie' were most subject to it.

By the later-seventeenth century, although its physical origin was not in dispute, the mental symptoms were considered more important than the fits: 'their Minds are more affected than their Bodies; for an incurable Desperation is mixt with the very nature of the Disease'.[20]

Nevertheless women not only had 'the vapours' in common

parlance for a long time to come, but some even still believed in the literal rising of the womb: 'That the Mother (as they call it) gets into the throat of married women and Maids, is by thousands believed to be a truth; yea, that the string of the Mother is fast in the throat'.[21]

The physical symptoms included in the fit, the cessation of movement and respiration, coldness and stiffness of the body, led to the belief that women might be buried alive in these fits. Paré mentioned a case in Spain where the puzzling and sudden death of a woman made her friends ask for an autopsy to find the cause, whereupon she came to life again at the first incision 'to the horrour and admiration of all the spectators'. Dr Chamberlain said 'doubtlesse many are buried in such fits, (for they last sometimes twenty four hours or more, and the bodies grow cold and rigid like dead Carkasses) who would return if time were waited on, and means used', and he advised that burial of such women should be delayed two or three days.[22] The kind of 'means used' were the logical result of what were believed to be the causes. The cure of the fits was chiefly aimed at drawing the uterus down into its proper place, evacuating superabundant seed, repressing filthy vapours from the head, and stirring up the spirits.

Although the literal rising of the womb could hardly have been accepted by Harvey, he mentioned two cases of hysterical women, one of whom was 'wilde by reason of a *Uterine Melancholy* and *Distemper*, for above ten years together', who were both cured quite fortuitously when they developed prolapse.[23] Most authors were persuaded that the best way to bring down the uterus and discharge the seed was by sexual intercourse: 'there is nothing better than for the man to anoint the top of his Yard with a little oil of Gilliflowers and oil of sweet Almonds together, and so to lie with her; for this assuredly brings down the Matrix again'.[24]

Where this was not practicable it was recommended that a midwife should dip her fingers in aromatic oils 'and then put them into the mouth of the matrice, rubbing it, long and easilie, that through that prouoking, the grosse and clammy humour may be auoided out'.[25] Not unnaturally there was some doubt whether this course of action was quite unexceptionable, morally speaking, a scruple which Culpeper considered foolish Popish superstition. But Ferrand, writing in 1640, complained that 'some Physitians . . . although they are Christians . . . doe notwithstanding prescribe for the cure of this disease, Lust, and Fornication'. He did not object to prescribing marriage, which Harvey did with complete success in a case of hysterical anaesthesia in a virgin in St Thomas's Hospital.[26]

For preventing the vapours ascending to the head a girdle made of the skin of a hart killed in the act of copulation was said to be effective. Riverius thought that if an ordinary swathe-band were tied tightly above the navel, the womb would be thereby reduced, and the vapours hindered from ascending. If the vapours should notwithstanding succeed in ascending to the head, 'The braine is so opprest sometimes that wee are compeld to burne the outward skin of the head, with hot oyle, or with a hot iron'.[27]

Various measures, some of the milder of which remained in common use in Victorian times, were used to stir up nature, such as cupping, rubbing the extremities with salt, vinegar and mustard, 'pulling the hairs of the privities with violence' and applying strong smells to the nose.

In the time of the actual fit 'we must presently make use of Hysteric Medicines, which by their strong and offensive smell, recall the disorderly and deserting Spirits to their proper Stations'.[28] Spirit of hartshorn, assa foetida, spirit of sal ammoniac, 'and whatever else has a filthy and ungratefull smell' were all suitable. For a shift one could burn feathers, hair, old shoes, tobacco, snuff, or a musket match, or 'you may hold a chambre vessell with old vrine to their nose'. Also highly esteemed was a fume made of 'the warts which grow upon Horses Legs; which being dried in an Oven, and beaten to Pouder, they are burnt under the Noses of women in these fits as a present Remedy, whereby women are wont to be in an instant delivered of their fits, to the admiration of the by-standers'.[29] The classic throwing cold water on the patient was mentioned, but some thought this was only safe if done in summer, the sun being in the tropic of cancer.

Prolapse required exactly the opposite treatment, since here the uterus needed to be put up rather than drawn down. But it too might arise from sexual frustration, 'a longing desire that oftentimes women have for the society of a man', as well as from humoral causes, hard childbirth and poor midwifery.

Attempts were made to cure the problem by medicines, chiefly drying and astringent fomentations, made for example from a healthy man's urine, and by fumigations to the womb of evil-smelling things. Several authors recommended advancing on the prolapse with a hot iron as if to burn it, which would frighten it in, or on the same principle placing mice tied by the tails or some other creeping vermin between the woman's thighs.

But the best surgeons used purely mechanical means. The prolapsed part was softened with oil and reduced by hand, or using a candle or a blunt stick padded with rag. Once returned to its normal place a pessary was inserted to support it, and a lengthy period of bed rest advised while it settled back in. The pessaries were usually made of boxwood or of cork sealed with wax. Sometimes they had a string attached to take them out for cleaning, or to fasten them to a girdle if they had a tendency to keep falling out. The round ones were supposed to be five or six inches in circumference, but many practitioners found the triangular ones with rounded corners stayed in better. Surgeons were advised to keep three or four of these handy, and some evidently did; Willughby, for example, saw a patient at St Thomas's Hospital in 1659 suffering from 'a great lapsus uteri, as big as two fists. I put it up . . . and, having about mee an uterine pessary . . . I conveyed the same presently into vagina uteri'. This enabled the patient to go about and do light work.[30] Where these pessaries were successful, 'the women notwithstanding do all their usuall enployments, conveniently are enjoyed by Men in carnal conjunctions, do conceive, carry their big Bellies, and bring forth'.[31] Sound instructions were given to support the prolapse manually when such women were in labour, if necessary leaving an assistant to receive the child.

Sometimes when treatment had been neglected the prolapsed part became so fouled with excrements that it became ulcerated or even gangrened, and was surgically removed by the knife, cautery or ligature. There was much dispute whether in these cases the whole womb was cut out, or merely a section of vaginal tissue. McMath said that some authors denied the possibility of total inversion, 'admitting only some laxity of the *Neck* or *Sheath*, which thus comes out and turns, hanging down like a Man's *Yard*, or a *Pudding*'.[32] This was the opinion of Van Roonhuyse, because, as he thought, the womb was up to two inches thick at term. But Mauriceau, who did not think the womb grew thicker in pregnancy, said that a total procidentia could occur, but only at a delivery, when the cervix was greatly widened.

Sharp asserted 'the whole womb may be taken forth when it is corrupted, as I have seen, and yet the woman may live in good health', but obviously this cannot be taken at face value when she says of another case in 1520, 'and that woman did afterward follow her ordinary business, and as she and her Husband confest and reported, she kept company with her husband, and cast forth Seed in Copulation, and had her monthly courses as she was wont to have before'.[33] Although most authors were inclined to believe it, Dionis at least doubted whether a total hysterectomy had ever so far actually been done.

Chlorosis, a type of severe anaemia characterised by extreme pallor, was considered to arise from obstructions: 'It may be defined thus: An evil habit of Body from the Obstruction of the Veins of the Liver, Spleen, and Mesentery, and especially of those which are about the Womb'.[34] The symptoms included a greenish pallor, breathlessness, tiredness and longings for 'Oatmeal, or ashes, or such ill trumpery'. By eating such things, and especially by drinking vinegar, the vessels were contracted and the humours vitiated, and thus the whole passage of the blood was hindered. If taken in time in young virgins it could be cured by marriage. Parents should therefore 'prudently and timely provide marriage for them; much of the Cure of this disease lying in Carnal Copulation, as experience hath and doth teach every day'.[35]

If this was not done and the disease advanced so far that the menses stopped, a very complicated course of physic became necessary involving bleeding, steel medicines, purging and so forth. Pale complexions of course were fashionable, and Maubray claimed some women, considering fresh-complexioned women mere rustics, not only did not seek to cure the pallor of the greensickness, but actually used means to turn their own complexions equally pallid.[36]

Yet another alarming disease arose through ungratified desire, 'and to such a height does the malady reach in some, that they are believed to be poisoned, or moon-struck, or possessed by a devil'.[37] This disease was called 'womb fury' and was sometimes taken to be a variant of hysteria, caused by unevacuated seed. According to Dr Chamberlain, maidens at puberty begin 'to think upon . . . *&c* [sic] for want whereof some pine away, and dwinder into Consumptions, others more vigorously rage, affected with the *Furor uteri*'.[38]

Riverius was particularly expansive upon the subject: 'Womb-Furie is a sort of Madness, arising from a vehement and unbridled desire of Carnal Imbracement, which desire disthrones the Rational Facul[t]y so far, that the Patient utters wanton and lascivious Speeches, in all places, and companies, and having cast off all Modesty, madly seeks after Carnal Copulation, and invites men to have to do with her in that way'. It chiefly affected virgins and young widows, 'although it may also betide married Women, that have impotent Husbands, or such as they do not much affect, whereby their Seminary Vessels are not sufficiently disburthened'. Marriage again where possible was prescribed: 'it is very good Advice in the Beginning of the Disease, before the Patient begins manifestly to rave, or in the space between her fits, when she is pretty well, to marry her to a lusty yong man. For so the Womb being satisfied, and the offensive Matter contained in its

Vessels being emptied, the Patient may peradventure be cured'.

Failing this, 'some advise that the Genital Parts should be by a cunning Midwife so handled and rubbed, as to cause an Evacuation of the over-abounding Sperm'. But Riverius, being a Papist, thought this was somewhat immoral, and that it might be enough to rub the belly, not touching the privy parts, while the patient was in the bath, so as to let in water to cool the womb.[39]

The symptoms of many gynaecological diseases mentioned in the textbooks were so circumscribed within the framework of humoral pathology that there is little possibility of translating them into recognisable diseases as we now see them. Such were the cold, moist, hot or windy distempers of the womb, the humoral inflations and dropsies, and many more.

In some cases a group of diseases can be roughly identified however. 'The whites', the pox and gonorrhoea form such a group. 'The whites' was a blanket term for almost any disease producing a vaginal discharge: it thus overlapped with gonorrhoea and the pox, and probably included all sorts of infective and ulcerative conditions. It was described as a flowing of excrementitious humours: 'And the said Excrementitious Humors are somtimes white and flegmatick, very like to Whey, or Barley Cream; somtime they are pale, or yellow, or green by the mixture of Choller; somtimes watery by the admixture of serous Humors: somtimes blackish, by the admixture of Melancholly; somtimes sharp and Corrosive, so as to eat into, and exulcerate some parts of the Womb; somtimes they are of a strong and beastly smel, and other whiles again, not at all offensive in that kind'.[40]

Gonorrhoea was often included in this class of diseases, and was believed to be simply what the name literally means, 'running of seed'. Since women and men both had seed, they could both suffer from involuntary shedding of seed. Some thought gonorrhoea was caused by 'venereal imaginations, and only happens in the time of sleep', and was thus much the same as nocturnal pollutions. Others thought it was peculiar to unchaste women and therefore, unlike the whites, a true venereal disease.

The French pox, however, included all the venereal diseases as we know them rolled into one, for even at the end of the eighteenth century it was still not established whether syphilis and gonorrhoea were one disease or two. In our period gonorrhoea might or might not be a symptom of the lecher's pox, but it might also develop into it if it acquired further malignity.

Ulcers of the womb and vagina might be due to the pox,[41] or to quite unrelated conditions, as might itching and inflammation. Lesions were divided into gentle and venemous, of which the latter were said to be contagious. However the division was more a matter of distinguishing degrees of severity and a more or less hopeful prognosis, than a statement about aetiology.

This also seems to have been true of tumours. Cancer was known from Hippocratic times, and was fairly well recognised clinically, at least in more accessible parts of the body such as the breast, and in its more advanced stages. It was classed as an inflammation of cold cause, of which a 'schirrus' was the usual forerunner. 'It is more evidently distinguished by the eye-sight, when it may be seen, as in the Neck of the Womb it may be, with the help of a Womb-perspective Instrument, for we shal see an uneven and bunching swelling, Lead-colored or black, compassed about with certain branches of Veins, as it were with roots.'

'A Cancer is a hard swelling of the Body or Neck of the Womb, which resists the touch, and causeth a most vehement pain, as it were pricking and cutting the part affected. It is caused by black Choller gathered in that part, or by reason of a Scirrhus, or senceless hard tumor il cured, which easily turns into a Cancer, especially in this part of the Body, by reason of the copious afflux of blood, which being retained in those Veins which are nigh unto the Scirrhus, and not sufficiently evacuated by the monthly purgations, it becomes adust or burned, and acquires a malignant disposition'.[42]

A cancer might thus be caused by empirics who 'administring to an inflammation of the wombe, doe over much refrigerate & astring the humour, that it can neither passe forward nor backward; hence the matter being condenst degenerates as it were into lapidious or hard substance'.[43]

Despite the firm belief that all cancers were incurable, remedies were proposed, notably frogs washed and boiled, and laid on as a poultice, or their broth used as an injection. Operative treatment was sometimes advised, not for cancers in the womb or vagina, which were generally treated by medical means, but for breast cancers, and for the king's evil in the breasts.

Sometimes it was proposed to extirpate only the obviously affected glands, but even this was often understandably more than the patient could face. Pechey recounted such a case, of a woman whose breast was ulcerated, 'but very hard *Glands* lay within, and in the circumference of the *tumour*, there were some *tubercles* that required to be eradicated; to which purpose, he [the surgeon] design'd to have slit open the *abscess*, and to have pull'd away the Cancerated *Glands*, but she would not permit him so much as to enlarge the orifice; upon which consideration he left her, and she died within half a year after'.[44]

Perhaps she was wise; Dr Richard Kay, assisted by his father, amputated the cancerous breast of a Mrs Driver of Crawshawbooth on 22 December 1748. She survived the operation, but by the following June the cancer had started to grow again, and the heroic Mrs Driver came to see the doctor determined to undergo a second operation, and had a large number of tumours dissected out from below the old scar and down into the abdomen. Similar operations followed in July, August, September and October; but on 20 February 1750, just over a year after the original mastectomy, Dr Kay attended Mrs Driver's funeral.[45]

But in most cases, perhaps more realistically, palliation of the pain only was attempted, with the only effective narcotic then known: 'I have seen a woman, having a Cancer in her Dug, that took every night for four months together, two or three grains of Laudanum, and had no hurt, but very great comfort thereby'.[46]

*Chapter Ten*

# Normal Childbirth

It is clear that labours varied very much in severity, not only necessarily, as a result of physical factors, but also because of differences in management and in the patient's attitude and expectations. The attitudes of patient and attendants were in good measure conditioned by social class.

It was generally assumed among people of the social classes who would call on professional attendants of repute, and who might be expected to know about and to demand the most modern and best treatment (best in the sense of what was *believed* best by the members of those social classes and their professional attendants) that childbirth was always painful and often dangerous. But it was also believed that nothing like the same pain and danger attended childbirth among other classes. Sometimes the hardy Scots or the wild Irish were said to have almost painless labours, sometimes working countrywomen, sometimes whores and doxies, who being accustomed to brutality and harshness, set light by the pain and peril of childbirth. Sometimes the known fact that women pregnant with bastards seemed often able to give birth unattended, without any screaming and groaning, get rid of the child, and return immediately to their usual work was described as evidence that the lower orders fared better in childbirth than the rich and respectable.

The obvious inference that patient expectation conditioned to a large extent the perception of childbirth as a painful, dramatic and dangerous process, or the reverse, was probably drawn first by Dr Grantley Dick-Read.[1] It was equally obvious that the differences in management between the childbed of the rich and the poor accounted to some extent for the apparent anomaly that the poor had their children more easily and reared them more successfully than the rich. But though this might have been suspected by some practitioners it was not until Charles White condemned the whole current approach to lying-in as unhealthy and productive of poor results that changes began to be made.[2] The factors militating against the earlier adoption of more rational methods of management were complex, and can only be mentioned here, but they included the 'mystique' of female traditional habits in childbirth; the social and psychological needs of pregnant women; the inter-professional jealousies and self-interest of midwives and men-midwives as groups; and the slow pace of scientific advance itself before the nineteenth century.

Obstetrics did of course change profoundly between the sixteenth and the eighteenth centuries, two of the most obvious changes being the invention of the obstetric forceps, and the irruption of men into midwifery practice. It is not so certain that the result was altogether an improvement. The ignorant, harsh and vulgar midwife who first appeared as a verbal cartoon figure in this period was sometimes replaced by the licentious, instrument-happy, self-serving man-midwife who also appeared as a cartoon figure a little later. Bad practitioners of both sexes existed throughout the period, as did good ones of both sexes. Bad practice existed alongside good, but it was not simply a question of class or sex. Indeed in obstetrics one step forward has not infrequently proved to be two steps back in the longer view.

The conduct of labour and birth described in the textbooks was thought to be the best modern management for those with means to obtain the best. Authors' opinions varied a good deal in points of detail, and views changed with time, but their comments on the habits of other social orders enable us to form a fair idea of what was actually done at various social levels and at different times.

Jonas considered the state of midwifery in his time to be bad enough to afford ample warrant for the publication of a textbook in English, however open to objection it might be on grounds of propriety. His much-quoted comment 'as touchynge mydwyfes, as there be many of them ryght expert, dilige*n*t, wyse, circumspecte, and tender aboute suche busynesse: so be there agayne manye mo full vndyscreate, vnreasonable, chorleshe, & farre to seke in suche thynges . . . Throughe whose rudenesse and rasshenesse onely I doubte not, but that a greate nomber are caste awaye and destroyed' was probably a fair estimate of the contemporary situation.[3] His own advice however in some respects seems to have contributed to a fall in the standards of midwifery during the next hundred years. Much of this advice, and still more the ignorant and over-zealous application of it, was gradually rejected by the writers on midwifery of the next century, but the damage done was not easily repaired.

Midwives were urged to handle the genital parts, stretch and dilate them, cut the membranes when they appeared or break them with their nails, urge the patient to go up and down stairs for an hour 'crying or reaching so loude as she ca*n*', then when sitting in the birth stool, bear down while the midwife pressed on the belly 'gently' to push the child downwards. Many prescriptions were given to affect the course of labour, and the midwife was told to extract the placenta immediately after the birth by pulling on the cord.

It is not possible to say how many of these ideas were new, since we know very little of mediaeval midwifery, but they certainly involve more physical interference with the patient than *Trotula*, where medicines and amulets are chiefly relied on. Thus *The birth of mankind* encouraged, or perhaps even initiated, the 'haling' midwifery so much complained of in the later seventeenth century.

The methods of managing difficult labours advised in it were already outmoded. Medicines were still much relied on to expel dead births, stir up flagging pains, support the spirits, expel the placenta, arrest bleeding, and so forth. Midwives seem to have given cordials, usually alcoholic, very freely, and the midwife's powder, given to promote the pains and expel the birth, was in ordinary use in the seventeenth century. By the eighteenth century the men-midwives had largely abandoned these ineffective remedies, but the female midwives continued the old ways, and were accused of getting their patients drunk as well as bullying them by forcing them to go up and down stairs, and by needlessly stretching and pulling the parts.

But these methods were either initiated by *The birth of mankind* or promoted by it, and it was probably therefore the better educated and more consciously professional midwife who learned them. Willughby came across many examples of this meddlesome midwifery, which in his early days he also regarded as good management, until experience of labour managed by less interfering methods convinced him that these practices were actually the cause of many painful and tedious labours, and the reverse of helpful.

The midwives Willughby described fell into two groups; those, often the young ones, who had read a little in a midwifery book and imagined they knew everything, and who at labours busied themselves with constant urging of the pains, stretching the parts and harrassing the patient; and those who, with less learning and less self-importance, contented themselves with chatting as they sat by, administering food and drink at intervals, and merely receiving the child as it was born. Some of these midwives did not even fetch the placenta, with successful results, but Willughby thought that was carrying non-interference too far.

If the case was clearly not normal these latter midwives did not trust to their own skills, but sent for a man-midwife. In such cases Willughby reported that his task was far easier than where the midwife had struggled on by herself, using the methods advised in *The birth of mankind*, and had thereby much worsened the situation before he was sent for.

On the psychological management of labour however, *The birth of mankind* gave good advice. The midwife was to support the patient, not only with food and drink, 'but also with swete wordes, geuynge her good hope of a spedefull delyueraunce, encouragyng and enstomacking her to pacience and tolleraunce'. Startlingly modern was the implicit recognition that labour falls into stages, during the first of which, while the cervix gradually dilates, nothing can be achieved by bearing down: 'But this must the mydwyfe aboue all thynges take hede of that she co*m*pell not the woman to labor, before the byrth come forewarde & shewe it selfe. For before that tyme all labor is in vayne, labor as muche as ye lyst. And in this case many tymes it cometh to passe, that the partie hath labored so sore before the tyme, that when she sholde labor in dede, her myght and strength is spent before in vaine, so that she is not nowe able to helpe her selfe, and that is a peryllous case'.[4] This was in practice familiar to the best men-midwives by Mauriceau's time, who mentioned a certain experienced man-midwife who used to sleep in an adjacent room during the first stage of labour, and 'never awaked till just the Child was in the passage, at which time the Woman changeth her moans to loud cries'.[5] Although repeated by others this particular piece of advice was not much heeded, and the ' 'ang on yer pains dearie' approach of many midwives in the early years of the present century, before the untrained pre-1902 midwives ceased to practice, is well remembered by the few remaining old ladies who encountered them.

Women themselves, moreover, often did not realise that their meddlesome midwives were incompetent. Willughby examined a patient whose midwife's violence had made a recto-vaginal fistula so that the woman voided her excrements through the vagina, 'yet this woman did much commend her laborious midwife, and said that shee took great paines to deliver her, to save her life'.[6] Women were naturally inclined to make much of these dangers and difficulties, and to vie with each other in reporting them. In 1793 Blunt complained that the women at confinements were too prone to terrify the patient with dismal tales about bad labours.[7] Thus bad practitioners escaped censure. And Dionis pointed out that 'an easy and sudden Delivery is not so much for a Woman's Reputation, especially in her first Child; for People are apt to conclude, that the Parts have been open'd and relax'd before, and therefore most Women are proud of being long in Labour'.[8]

It was an often repeated belief that 'poor Women, Hirelings, Rusticks, and others us'd to hard Labours, also Viragoes, and Whores, who are clandestinely delivered, bring forth without great difficulty, and in a short time after, rising from their Bed, return to their wonted Labours: but Women that are rich, tender and beautiful, and many living a sedentary Life, as tho they partak'd of the Divine Curse after a more severe manner, *bring forth in Pain*, and presently after their delivery lye in an uneasie and dangerous condition'.[9] Hard and dangerous labour thus acquired a social cachet, and much assiduous attendance seemed essential for women of quality. Practitioners no doubt found this idea useful to increase their own importance, and hence their fees.

Pechey was by no means alone in advocating totally different treatment in childbed, especially after the delivery, for different social classes: 'for she that thinks to order an ordinary labouring, or Country-woman, like a person of quality, kills her, and she that thinks to govern a person of quality like an ordinary Country-woman, does the same to her'.[10]

Many midwives did not even know enough to examine the patient and ensure she was really in labour, but as soon as they were called bestirred themselves with exhortations to bear down, and with stretching the parts. Willughby often advised patients not to permit such interference, but those who were not over-ruled by the midwife often found themselves regarded as peevish and unmanageable by her. Sudell said women often suffered from the ignorance of these midwives, especially young inexperienced mothers, 'who think they are bound, and that it is their wisdom to do as the good wives bid them, and its common amongst them though but stragling, degenerate and wild pains, to bid them stop their mouths, hold their breath, and strain downwards'.[11] Advice to the midwife to stretch the parts, and to cut the membranes, was still given in 1671 by Mrs Sharp, while another author writing in the same year strongly disapproved of both practices.[12] Stretching the parts, though much opposed by Willughby, was still thought permissible if carefully done, by Read. Pressing down the belly on the other hand, which Willughby did not condemn, Read, following

Mauriceau, thought did more harm than good.

Most good midwives gave a clyster early in labour, both to make more room for the head, and to prevent the excrements coming away involuntarily during the birth. They also ensured the patient's bladder was emptied, and used a silver catheter if need be. Some thought a wide swathe-band passed under the woman's back and lifted up equally on both sides by assistants as the pains came was helpful. It was usual to conduct the delivery in a darkened room, with a blazing fire. Practitioners had a dread of cold entering the womb, and needless uncovering of the patient was condemned, both for this reason and for modesty's sake. It was common for a large number of female neighbours and friends to be present, two might hold down the patient's shoulders, two more grip her hands, two might be busy with the swathe-band, others pressing down the belly, others offering drink or medicine, and the midwife in the midst of it all stretching and anointing the parts.

*The birth of mankind* recommended that the actual delivery should take place on the birth-stool, which was illustrated and described in detail. It seems the birth-stool was not then familiar to English readers; Jonas said birth-stools were in use 'in some regio*n*s (as in France and Germanye)'.[13] However according to Willughby the London midwives used them when he lived there about a century later, and they were apparently still occasionally used in the eighteenth century.[14] By then however they were out of fashion in France, following the advocacy of bed delivery by Guillemeau and others. By Mauriceau's time, in 1660, at the Hôtel Dieu, the women were delivered in a special bed in a room called 'the stove', and then walked to the recovery wards. By the turn of the eighteenth century, Dionis regarded birth-stools as an English idea, which although they had advantages would be difficult to introduce in France.

Willughby disapproved of the birth-stool and preferred the newer French idea of delivery in bed for normal births. Probably in country districts in England where the midwives did not have stools, women were delivered on a bed, on the floor, on an assistant's lap, standing leaning on a table, and even kneeling on all fours. Delivery in a kneeling position was said to be common in country districts. It was very unusual in England for the husband to be present, and remained so until very recently, though Sudell thought it could be done with advantage where the woman wished it and the husband was of the right temperament.

By the end of the seventeenth century bed delivery was normal except among the poorest and most rural women, and the lithotomy position was the commonest. In the books emphasis was put upon 'keeping touch with the Mothers Endeavours' and 'drawing forth the Child when 'tis upon the move' rather than trying to force nature.

Throughout the time it was believed vital to extract the placenta immediately after the birth, for fear the cervix should close and prevent its exclusion, when it would putrefy and set up dangerous symptoms. Where the woman had no attendants, or only friends, the placenta would probably be left to come itself. Although some midwives allowed it to be excluded naturally it was universally deemed better practice and proof of greater skill, if the midwife or man-midwife 'fetched' it.

*The birth of mankind* advised simply pulling the cord, albeit warning that it must be done gently. This same method was advised also by Mauriceau, but he described assisting by manual external pressure on the abdomen in addition. Willughby advised simply gathering the placenta in the hand when it descended into the vagina, and he also favoured the expulsion of clots and retained products by external manual expression, either by the woman herself, or by an experienced nurse-keeper.[15] Although Harvie, in the mid-eighteenth century, preferred to let the placenta come by itself, he found patients demanded its extraction.[16]

Despite the warning in *The birth of mankind* to use traction on the cord gently, unfortunate accidents sometimes resulted from the use of this method. Indeed Maubray went so far as to say 'Nothing is more common among ignorant unwary MIDWIVES, than to *invert* and *draw down* the *Bottom* of the WOMB itself, by pulling the *Navel-String*, as they foolishly intend by *means* of it only to extract the SECUNDINE'.[17]

In the late seventeenth century it was suggested, particularly by Deventer, that a better method was to introduce the whole hand promptly into the uterus and by sweeping it round to clear the womb both of placenta and retained debris. This method, it was further claimed, prevented the error of extracting a twin placenta unawares before the delivery of the second twin, ensured that nothing praeternatural like a mole was in the womb, and enabled the practitioner to satisfy himself that the womb was contracting properly, and had not become displaced.[18] Read also favoured manual removal, but was careful to add that it was better 'to leave some part of it behind, than to scrape or scratch the least part of the Womb, for fear of a Flooding, Inflammation, or Gangrene, which cause death'.[19]

Since no-one as yet had any notion of aseptic procedures this practice was thought very safe, and was recommended to midwives. 'A Midwife, who is not thus careful to introduce her Hand, but only takes what comes away of itself, may probably leave something behind, to the great Peril and Prejudice of the Woman. The remaining Pains are oftentimes imperfect, and so pass under the Denomination of *After-Pains*, till a bad *Fever* is kindled, or *Floodings* are occasioned; Both which generally prove fatal, and might have been prevented by this Method, which was also *Daventer's*, as may be seen in his Treatise, and which I believe is the present Practice of the greatest Masters in the Profession. Nor are the Examples of many Women doing very well, under the Management of such Midwives, as never to pass [sic] the Hand, any Objection to this Method, since No one was ever hurt by it, but Thousands on the contrary have suffered, nay died, by the Omission thereof.'[20]

Barret pointed out that the manual extraction of the placenta, properly done, enhanced the midwife's reputation: 'the Company is generally curious to see it, and if it be whole, not torn, or rent, it redounds to the credit and reputation of the Midwife. Therefore I would advise all Midwives never to extract the Burthen, without putting up their Hand to separate it cleanly from the Womb'.[21]

A number of midwives' customs and beliefs about the birth were already regarded as old wives' tales by the seventeenth century. The belief that a child born in a caul would be fortunate, or according to others unfortunate, was all but universal, and the caul was often dried and preserved in a box, although others warned midwives never to keep the caul for sorcerers to make use of. The notion was dismissed as 'Old *Wifes* Frivolous *Clatters*, or Crafty *Fictions* some *Midwifes* uses to amuse silly Credulous *People*', by most writers, although Mrs Sharp admitted to a belief in it.

The navel-string was also sometimes dried and a piece put in a ring as a protection against the falling sickness, convulsions, witches and devils. We have already seen that it was thought the navel-string, when cut, influenced the size of the penis; according to Guillemeau 'to speake the truth, the Gossips commonly say merrily to the Midwife; if it be a boy, *Make him good measure*; but if it be a wench, *Tye it short*'. This idea passed from a scientific fact to an old wives' tale within our period. Foretelling by the number and spacing of the knots on the cord the number of future children, on the other hand, was treated as dubious and ridiculous in the textbooks, though it seems to have been current. Midwives also believed that the longer the cord took to fall off the longer the child would live, and that if the cut end was allowed to touch the ground the child would never hold its water. All this made cutting the string an important matter, and a test of the midwife's skill.[22]

To stimulate a weak child it was usual to put the placenta in hot wine, in the belief that the vapour would be imbibed through the cord, but this practice also became regarded as superstitious by the late-seventeenth century. Nevertheless men-midwives were advised not to forbid it, though useless, or the bystanders would feel a necessary measure had been neglected. Another method of reviving the child was to stroke back into its body the blood in the cord before cutting it. Willughby approved of this, but by the end of the seventeenth century it had come to be thought bad practice, in case the blood had become chilled and clotted. It has been shown in modern studies however that a significant percentage of blood can be restored to the circulation by this method.

The vernix on the child's body was believed by some women 'of easie belief' to be cream cheese, because they had often eaten some when they were with child. The placenta was generally thrown away or buried, since some people thought it dangerous to burn it: 'Those who pretend to explain things by Sympathy, forbid us to throw the After-Burden into the Fire. 'Tis an easy matter to gratify 'em in this, and it is but fit we should; for if the Womb happens to be inflam'd, tho we point out the Cause of it with the greatest Certainty, yet they will hear of no other than *that*'.[23] It evidently did not pay a practitioner to scoff at these female superstitions too openly, however ridiculous he might think them. According to Sharp, though some had tried to make use of the placenta in medicine it was usually thrown away, but McMath thought this was unfortunate, since volatile salt extracted from the placenta was particularly efficacious in expediting delivery.

The management of lying-in differed even more from modern practice than the actual birth, at least among the well-to-do. After the birth the woman was kept warm to a degree of perceptible perspiration. Guillemeau directed 'the doores, and windows of her chamber in any wise are to be kept close shut'. It was believed that the eyesight was much weakened by labour, and the room was kept dark for at least three days.

It was considered excellent practice to wrap the belly in a sheepskin freshly flayed off, and according to some also in the skin of a hare flayed alive, and then its throat cut and the blood rubbed on the skin. The flayed sheepskin was still much commended in the eighteenth century. Chapman declared 'I have for many Years past had a happy Experience of this Method, and wish I had come sooner to the Knowledge of it than I did, as having always employed it with Success'.[24] Mauriceau regarded it as 'a remedy of too much trouble; for there must always be a Butcher ready for every Woman that is laid, or some other person that can do it as readily, who must for this purpose be in the very Chamber, or at least in the House, that so they may have the skin very hot according to directions'.[25] Poeton objected to it because after two or three days 'the smell thereof . . . woulde much annoy the woman, and all that shoulde com neare her, as experience hath manifested in other cases'; usually however the skin was only left on for an hour or two. There always remained the possibility that much alarm might be caused to the assembled ladies, should the sheep pursue the butcher into the room, as Dionis said it did on the occasion of the Dauphiness' first confinement. After the sheepskin was removed elaborate bolstering and swathing of the belly was usual, to squeeze out the lochia and to settle the womb back into its proper place. Mauriceau complained that nurse-keepers swathed so tightly they tended to suppress the lochia rather than promote them. He believed however that the woman ought to lie completely still, flat on her back, to prevent the womb becoming displaced, whereas Willughby said that this was a notion of foolish nurses, and no harm could possibly come of a woman lying whichever way she felt most comfortable. Some midwives on the ninth day after a woman's delivery enjoined her very strictly to lie still on her left side, by which means they claimed the womb was resettled in its proper place.[26]

The newly delivered woman was generally given a drink to sooth the throat made of two ounces of syrup of maidenhair and two of oil of sweet almonds, but it made some women so sick that it did them more harm than good. Some were said to take 'two drops of the *blood* which comes out of the Navel string of the Infant, and give it mingled to the Woman in the foresaid Syrups, though there is much fault to be found with this, by reason of the nastiness of it'.[27]

Cleansing the parts with a herbal decoction was usual, though some women used barley water and some milk. Others found milk unsuitable, because although it was soothing it curdled and became offensive. Portal favoured salt water, but his patients with minor lacerations must have found it trying.

The textbooks ordered absolute rest and quiet for some days after the birth, and much condemned the common practice of making a celebratory 'upsitting' on the third or fourth day, often coinciding with a noisy and bibulous christening party. This they thought did harm all sorts of ways; the cakes and pastries provided were bad for the patient, the presence of the company prevented her from using her bed-pan, and their noise and disturbance tended to over-tire her and bring on fevers. Although ordinary women got up about the third day the unanimous advice of authors was that the longer the woman stayed in bed the better, even up to a fortnight, a recommendation only feasible for leisured women.

It had at one time been the practice to keep the patient awake for some hours after the delivery, in the belief that sleep caused the natural heat to retire inwards and promoted haemorrhage, but at the end of the seventeenth century this was considered old-fashioned, and the patient was now directed to sleep in her dark, quiet, stuffy room.

If the woman was costive, clysters were advised, but on no account senna, of which, given by various unskillful women, 'some have been very ill, and others have died. For nature is now weakned, by the Travel, and while it is labouring to restore the body to its former Estate, is not to be disturbed with violent purgations'.[28]

As to diet, authors agreed that nurses, and women generally, had very erroneous ideas. Nurses urged the woman to feed plentifully to restore the blood she had lost, and even gave her oatmeal caudles, which the better informed knew were notably binding and gave women the greensickness. The correct diet was a low diet, as for wounded persons, consisting of jellies, gruel, broth and so on, and on no account flesh meat, which was far too feverish. Ordinary working women however had strong stomachs and could take more and stronger food than ladies of quality, and for them it might suffice to reduce their normal intake of food somewhat. But ideas on diet did vary, Portal used to let his lying-in patients have any food they liked, even meat, except just when the milk came in, and never found it did any harm.

A more ample diet could also be allowed to women who nursed their own children, which the rich almost never did. Not only did they have to adopt a restricted diet, they had to take other measures also to drive back the milk. Among such measures were fomentations of sage and box leaves boiled in urine; oil and vinegar, or a mixture of Galen's cooling ointment and populeum ointment, (both generally available at the apothecary's) spread on rag or brown paper and applied to the breasts. Willis said that the milk could be repelled by 'gently astringent Cere-Cloths, as with the red Lead Plaister *&c*'.

According to Mauriceau it was commonly believed highly effective for a woman 'to put on her Husbands shift yet warm, immediatly after he hath taken it off, and wear it until the Milk be gone: but in case the Milk doth in the mean time vanish, 'tis superstitious to believe that this Shirt is the cause of it . . . it happens rather, because all the humours of the Body of their own accord taking another course than to the Breasts, do not daily flow in so great abundance to them'.[29]

Dionis thought that most of the topical applications in vogue were also quite useless, but that it was not politic to neglect them: 'We must not be so credulous as to believe that a Linen-Rag dipt in any Liquor, and applied to the Breasts, will drive back the Milk, and change the ordinary Course of Nature. However, tho the Surgeon expects very little from such Applications, he must by no means omit them, for the satisfaction of conceited Women, who are apt to think themselves neglected, if something of this nature is not done, and will not fail to make loud Complaints of him, if they have any Disease of the Breasts afterward'.[30]

Since so many wealthy women refused to nurse their children, methods of repelling milk tend to feature more importantly in the textbooks than methods of establishing and improving breast-feeding, though it was universally considered that the best lactagogue was powdered earthworms. Nevertheless authors were generally agreed that women ought to nurse their own children. Pechey considered the many diseases of the breast which arose from suppressing the milk were a judgement on these unnatural mothers, and that only want of milk could be considered a just excuse.[31]

Wolveridge pointed out that rich women could nurse their children with less trouble than others, because servants could look after them in between. Much emphasis was put on the inadequacies of most wet-nurses. Sharp declared that 'The usual way for rich people is to put forth their children to nurse, but . . . it changeth the natural disposition of the child, and oftentimes exposeth the infant to many hazards'. She considered that mothers who did not nurse their own children never established a sound emotional bond with them, and that many women who claimed to be too delicate to nurse were really making excuses for want of natural affection.

Wet-nurses were accused of sluttishness and carelessness; they did not change the babies often enough or wash their clothes properly; they pretended to have more milk than they really had; they drank too much and overlaid the children; and they were too wanton and amorous; in short there was more abuse in nurses than in anything, 'for let them make what excuse they will, it is nothing but necessity that reduceth them to be such, although the greatest part do say that it is to get acquaintance'.[32] As a result of these abuses the children 'are sluttish or slovenly so long as they live; or else (being abused at nurse, are distort and Ricketty; full of botches, nasty, and nauseous to their own parents'.[33]

Although it was more usual to send the baby away to a nurse, often in the country, sometimes rich women took the nurse into their own household instead, so that the nurse was supervised, and so that by eating the same food as the mother 'the Child may suck the like milk with that which relieved it in the Mothers belly, or at least made of the same meats'. But another school of thought held that nurses accustomed to poverty, want and hardship yielded a firm milk, and that if they were taken into the household and well fed 'this makes the Milk rampant, the Child Humoursom'.

One had to be careful to choose a nurse whose own child was of the same sex, 'For the milk of a male child will make a female nursery more spritely, and a man-like Virago; and the milk of a girl will make a boy the more effeminate'.[34] Red-haired women made particularly bad nurses, because their milk was extremely hot. Some thought infants who had been nursed by red-haired women were especially liable to have the rickets, but no less an authority than Glisson did not entirely accept this.

Paré claimed that many husbands took such pity on their wives that they would not allow them to add the strain of nursing to that of bearing; but it is perhaps not cynical to suggest that they were more motivated by the general belief that during nursing, sexual intercourse was 'perfect venom to the milk' and must be foregone. Wolveridge went so far as to say that nurses must not even think about sex for fear that 'dreaming at night of that which their minds run on in the day, and by other filthy pollutions they infect the milk. So also, by the use of their husbands the Courses are stirred up, by which both the plenty and goodness of milk is derived another way; . . . or else the Nurse conceiveth with child, and so the infant becometh diseased and Ricketty, by sucking grumous, curdy, and unwholsome milk'.[35] Copulation diminished the milk, 'and maketh it of an unsavoury taste, tasting hot, and rank, or goatish'.[36] Maubray alone, in a rare fit of common sense, declared any clean healthy woman who ate sensibly could nurse satisfactorily, and could even have '*Conjugal Conversation*; notwithstanding the contrary Opinion of most *Authors*, provided only that she does not give the CHILD *suck* for an Hour or two after *Copulation*'.[37]

Good nurses of course never menstruated, and if this should happen must wean the child at once; indeed 'there dies a third part of the children, for want of taking care in this particular, which seem fat, and in good case'.[38] The prohibition of intercourse and the injunction to wean if menstruation should begin are easily explained by contemporary ideas about the physiology of lactation. This also underlay both the belief that the mother's milk was best, and also some curious ideas about the conduct of breast feeding during the puerperium.

The period of time during which the milk was considered unwholesome, partaking of the lochia and other humours voided after childbirth, varied from a day or two to a month, according to different opinions. Doubtless, working women paid little attention to such niceties, and Mauriceau admitted that some people even believed 'the Milk of a Woman new-laid is better at the beginning than when it is purified, and that it opens the Belly and purgeth the *Moeconion* from the Guts; but the gripes, which this overheated and foul Milk also causeth in him, is much more prejudicial than the good it otherwise doth'.[39] He favoured a delay of four or five days. Guillemeau preferred eight days or up to a month till the lochia ceased, 'In which space she shall let little prettie whelpes sucke her brests, to make her milke come the better, and that it goe not away. Some women do make their keepers draw their breasts, and others draw them with glasses themselves'.[40]

Sharp considered 'It is not good for a woman presently to suckle her child because those unclean purgations cannot make good milk, the first milk is naught'.[41] Maubray thought the infant should only have a little sugared wine two or three times a day until its stomach was cleared of phlegm, after which 'the *Breast* of some other clean and sound *Woman* may be given the CHILD, until the *Mother's Milk* be purified for its proper *Use*; which it can scarce be supposed to be . . . before the *ninth day* after DELIVERY'.[42]

In the meantime the baby had to have a wet-nurse, or be hand fed with pap, panada, and such substitutes, which were quite often given to very young babies, even when the mother herself nursed the child. La Vauguion indeed disapproved of giving pap to newborn babies, which he thought caused all sorts of problems, including convulsions, and might be fatal. In those unfortunate cases where no wet-nurse could be had, as for example when the child was poxed, he suggested expressing the nurse's milk into a porringer and spoon-feeding, or using a funnel of rolled rag to suck the milk through, though the best method was to let the child nurse from a young goat. It was an important man and a knight whose baby daughter was not allowed to suck a London nurse for fear of the pox, and was 'unfittingly nourished', evidently on pap and such substitutes, until at six days when a nurse endeavoured to feed her the child had forgotten how to suck, and so the poor thing died at ten days.[43]

No doubt the nursing practices of the less affluent and more ignorant women, who had no choice but to nurse their own children, compared favourably with those of the rich, just as their inability to provide the hot-house coddling then thought necessary for the wealthy during lying-in also did the poor an unintended favour; together these circumstances go a long way towards explaining the many cases of working women bearing and rearing children with an ease and success which much astonished the rich and their mentors.

*Chapter Eleven*

# The Management of Obstetric Complications

It was commonly observed that in a normal birth, nature alone would deliver the woman and only a little ordinary care was needed. It was also generally agreed that when anything abnormal occurred the case was potentially very dangerous, and much skill and knowledge was needed to avert disaster. But at the time *The birth of mankind* was published midwives had no effective way of dealing with even the commonest obstetric complications, and the woman laboured on until the birth — often of a dead child — finally occurred, or until she died undelivered. If the child was believed to be dead it might be delivered by hooked instruments to save the mother; apart from this kind of instrumental delivery however there were no techniques available that could be of any possible use.

Many measures were *believed* to be useful, including charms and medicines, and those cases which finally terminated in a spontaneous birth were very often credited to the successful use of such things, thus delaying the realisation that they were wholly ineffective, except perhaps psychologically.

Although in France better methods of dealing with some complications were being popularised among the surgeons, these methods were slow to be disseminated by the popular textbooks, and midwives were not willing to abandon faith in the medicines and other methods they traditionally used, so that quite late in the seventeenth century many writers contented themselves with prescriptions, and advice to call a man-midwife in desperate cases.

Many of the causes of painful and tedious labour were perfectly well recognised in Tudor times, such as extreme youth or age, weakness, apprehension and lack of fortitude in the mother, the excessive size of the child, or its presenting any way other than the normal vertex. Complications such as convulsions, haemorrhage and retained placenta were described also. There were in addition some accidental factors erroneously thought to cause bad labours, such as scent in the room, persons present crossing their fingers, or the patient forgetting to remove some amulet worn to prevent abortion.

Psychological factors were recognised; Barrough noted that the labour tended to be difficult if the mother were faint-hearted and intolerant of pain, and Paré said women were often hindered in labour by shyness because of the presence of a man, or by hatred to some woman present.

In all these cases, and often when more serious complications arose, expulsive or cordial medicines were relied on, and some people still had faith in such medicines in the eighteenth century, though the better obstetricians used them less and less. Mauriceau said mithridate and treacle ought not to be given to women in difficult labour, but rather good nourishment that would 'comfort the Stomach, without nauseating it, as those Drugs do which are only good for them that sell them'.[1]

Rueff gave prescriptions for two sorts of birth pills effective in procuring a speedy birth, which he said were approved by almost all the experts and were in use. Sermon's prescription ran 'Take Myrrh, Bay berries, the dryed Liver of Eles, of each one dram, beat them all into powder, and give it at twice in hot Sack. With this very Medicine I have helped many, when they have been in Labour four or five dayes in great misery . . . which by taking of this have been with ease delivered in less then one hour'.[2]

*The birth of mankind* recommended a fumigation of the dung or hoofs of an ass, and Sermon considered this fume of the most wonderful virtue. He also approved of giving the patient a good draught of her husband's urine, or bitches' milk, or the milk of another woman. Dr Chamberlain condemned this last remedy as a notion of '*Quacking Culpepper*', commenting 'There is little reason for it, and I am sure its loathsome to most women'. Willughby gave a prescription of his own for a birth powder which he claimed to have used successfully.[3] Pechey's birth powder contained savin leaves, cinnamon and saffron, and the same sorts of medicine were still recommended in *Aristotle's masterpiece*. So was the aetites stone; this stone was believed to draw out a dead child or a retained placenta as easily as the magnet draws iron, and solemn warnings were given to take it away again immediately after the birth, lest it should draw down the womb itself, its magnetic effect was so strong.[4]

Poor midwifery was often blamed for difficult labours in the seventeenth century. Despite the clear warning in *The birth of mankind* not to urge women to bear down too soon many midwives continued to do so, and made otherwise normal labours into tedious and difficult ones. Harvey complained that over-zealous midwives mismanaged cases. 'And therefore the younger, more giddy, and officious Midwives are to be rebuked; which, when they hear the woman in travaile, cry out for paine, and call for help; lest they should seem unskilful at their trade, and less busie then comes to their share, by daubing over their hands with oyles, and distending the parts of the *Uterus*, do mightily bestirre themselves, and provoke the expulsive faculty by medicinal potions: so that . . . by their desire to hasten and promote the Birth, they do rather retard and pervert it, and make it an unnatural and difficult delivery . . . and vainly perswading them [patients] to their three-legged stoole, weary them out, and bring them in danger of their lives'.[5]

Willughby was vehemently opposed to officious midwifery: 'let the midwife forbeare to use violence, which hindereth the birth, through much haling, or pulling, or stretching those tender parts. Such doings create paines, with swellings and sorenes, and make the labouring woman unwilling to endure her labour, and the putting down of her throwes; and, severall times, this too much officiousnes causeth evil accidents to follow, as tearing the body, sores, and ulcers, or flouding and scouring. All which, in childbed, bee found too oft dangerous, and they may prove fatall'.[6] He explicitly blamed these methods for some maternal deaths: 'in severall places, unto which I have beene sent for, I have found the mother undelivered, and shee and the child dead before I could come unto them, through the ignorance of such midwives'.[7] But Chapman in the early-eighteenth century still found that women had often been pressed into straining too soon, because the midwives could not tell by examination whether the time was right.[8]

The over-generous use of cordials by the midwives caused problems sometimes, as Giffard discovered: 'What in some measure occasioned the difficulty, was the Woman's being stupified and senseless from the quantity of strong liquors that was given her, and her smoaking Tobacco, so that she was very drunk, and no ways capable of pursuing directions, nor of assisting me by bearing down at the time of my extracting the Child'.[9]

Although *The birth of mankind* advised tearing or cutting the membranes if they did not break readily, Willughby condemned the practice as dangerous, and often the cause of the child not turning properly; but Pechey, in 1698, was still complaining of midwives who for haste to be gone to other women tore the membranes with their nails, thus endangering both mother and child.

When an obstetric emergency arose, whether through poor

management or unavoidably, there was a general agreement that midwives tended to send for help too late, either from failure to recognise the emergency, or unfounded confidence in their own capacities, so that the operative delivery of the child became much more difficult by the child's being wedged in the pelvis.

The malpresentation of the child was, as it still is, one of the commonest causes of abnormal labour. The problem was believed to be sometimes caused by the behaviour of the woman herself: 'The unseasonable motion of the Woman much retards the Delivery, as when she . . . flings her self about unadvisedly so that the Child cannot be Born the right way, being turned preposterously by the restlessness of the Mother'.[10] By the same reasoning it was for a long time suggested that the birth would right itself if the mother rolled about on her bed. According to Barrough many attendants resorted to shaking such patients violently. Willughby, who did not approve of this method, attended a case where the woman had been tossed in a blanket, which he found very shocking; in his view rolling the woman on the bed 'may casually alter the birth, but I beleeve, that it seldome, or never doth it'.

In *The birth of mankind*, and other early midwiferies, very complicated descriptions were given of every possible, and many impossible, postures in which the child could conceivably present. But the sole advice offered was to turn all such births to the head, first putting back any limbs that might be sticking out. Sensible as this advice sounded, it was not very practicable, as later authors pointed out: 'Most Authors advise . . . to change the figure, and place the Head so, as it may present first to the birth; but if they would shew how it should be done, we might follow their Counsel; which is very difficult, if not impossible to be performed'.[11] But even in 1698 Pechey, making no reference to podalic version, advised that where one foot presented the foot should be returned, 'which being done, let the woman rock her self from one side of the bed to the other . . .' till she apprehend the Child to be turned, upon which she may immediately expect her pains with all the assistance that may be given'.[12] Frequently also, even where midwives succeeded in forcing back the arm or foot which was protruding, they found the birth still unsuccessful. Willughby commented, 'my practice hath shewed mee, That, in severall of these births, through the midwives struglings to reduce the arme, that the arm hath been broken by them, and the child destroyed, and although, through much enforcement, they have reduced the arme, yet, through the woman's sufferings, and the midwife's strivings, the labouring woman hath been left so weak, that shee could not bee delivered by the midwife'.[13]

Although it was well known that in many of these difficult labours the woman's pains might go off, much faith was placed in medicines to provoke the expulsive faculty. Rueff's medicine, which he particularly favoured when the labour was obstructed and the pains failing, contained myrrh, cinnamon and saffron in pennyroyal water. In cases where uterine inertia set in and the patient was very faint, Sermon favoured a fume of white amber to smell. Only when such medicines had been tried and failed was it likely that operative delivery would be considered.

The problem of disproportion between the child's head and the pelvis was not well understood until the later seventeenth century; so long as it was believed the pelvic bones separated, or at least the ligaments stretched, it was assumed that the child could not be too big for the pelvis, but only for the cervix and vagina. Therefore the midwife thought the best way to help such a case was to be liberal in the use of oils and emollients, and to be more diligent in stretching and dilating the parts. Maubray said that where the ill position of the coccyx prevented the head bearing upon the cervix to distend it, 'most MIDWIVES (not knowing better) ascribe the whole *Difficulty* to the Orifice of the WOMB and the VAGINA; upon which they ignorantly fall a-tearing and dilating both the *One* and the *Other*'.[14] Even at the beginning of the eighteenth century, when pelvic inadequacy and deformity had come to be recognised as important causes of obstructed labour, Maubray found that nothing was more common, in cases where the pelvis was small and narrow, than for midwives to urge strong labour and give forcing medicines, although in his view the more slowly the birth proceeded the more readily the head would mould to the space available.

Although stitching of perineal tears was advocated in *Trotula* and instructions were given in *The birth of mankind* to sew such tears with silk 'as surgeons do other woundes', it does not seem that stitching such tears was common practice, either because of resistance on the part of the patient, or squeamishness on the part of the midwife. Realising this *The birth of mankind* offered an ingenious alternative: 'Take two lyttell peces of lynnen cloth, eche of the length of the wounde, & in bredth two fyngers brode: spred the lyttell clothes with some faste cleauynge plaster the which wyll cause the clouthes to stycke fast where they shalbe set, then fasten them the one on the one syde of the ryfte, the other on the other syde, so that nothyng appeare betwene the peces of lynnen in the myddes of them, but onely the clefte and ryfte of the wounde in the breadthe of a strawe, then this done, sowe these sydes of lynnen together close as before I bed you to sowe the skynne: & when they be thus stytched to gether, laye a lyttell lyquyd pytche vpon the seme: and this done the lappes and sydes of the wond vnder the lynnen plaster wyll grow to gether agayne & heale, & the*n* may ye remoue your plasters'.[15]

Some practitioners deliberately did not suture tears, so as to facilitate ensuing deliveries. Willughby advised that 'Where this grief can, without trouble bee suffered, it will bee much better not to meddle with it, then to endeavour to cure it. For it will cause the next labour to bee more dolorous, and difficult, by making a new laceration, or incision. But, not being cured, the ensuing births will bee more easy, by reason of the spaciousnes of the breach, the vulva and intestinum rectum being laid together, and making but one passage'.[16]

Severe perineal lacerations may have been not uncommon, partly because of the practice of stretching the parts, and partly through the use of instruments. Willughby mentioned more than one case where 'haling' midwives had made perineal tears extending to the anus, and Dr Chamberlain noted that after embryotomy 'sometimes it comes to pass, that by the violence of the extraction, the genitals of the Mother are so dilacerated, that urine, and excrements, which frequently happens, do involuntarily issue'.[17] Portal also thought such cases were too common, and de Venette said that 'Child-bearing is often accompanied with such dismal Accidents, that the women are torn after a surprizing rate. I have seen such as have had both holes in one'.[18] Yet if the parts did not heal together, despite the fact that the tear became 'a noysom *Latrin* for the future', the woman may have been fortunate rather than otherwise, since if the parts cicatrised together, although conception would not necessarily be impossible, the birth would be impossible, unless surgically-assisted or effected in the way described in a case Harvey quoted.[19] This concerned a woman 'who had all the interiour part of the neck of her *Womb* excoriated and torne, by a *difficult* and *painful delivery*' so that after it healed the whole genital tract was sealed up; yet she proved pregnant again, 'the time of her delivery being now arrived, the poor soul was lamentably tortured, and laying aside all expectation of being delivered, she resigned up her keys to her Husband, and setting her affairs in order, she took leave of all her friends. When behold, beyond expectation, by the strong contest of a very lusty Infant, the whole tract was forced open, and she was miraculously *delivered*'.[20]

It seems likely that unless the tear was too extensive to live with it was more usual to leave the cure to nature, or to use medicines only.

Dr Chamberlain did not suggest stitching, even where there was a total rent of the perineum, but proposed various medications, including an ointment made of oil of worms and foxes and a little blind whelp well boiled.

But Paré and most of the French men-midwives advised stitching, and suggested that the woman ought to be delivered in future by a man-midwife, since the same accident was almost impossible to avoid next time because of the rigidity of the scar. La Vauguion, although he admitted the scar would complicate the next delivery, nevertheless favoured stitching, because 'the Excrements coming that way disgust the Husband, and the Woman is by no means fit for his Caresses'.

Willughby considered a retained placenta 'will prove difficult and troublesome to the midwife to fetch, and few know how to do it, and they had better to let it alone unfetched, then to keep much strugling in the woman's body'.[21] This tended to happen especially where the cord had broken off in the attempt to extract a difficult placenta by traction. The medicines and methods for expelling the afterbirth advised in *The birth of mankind*, such as blowing hard into the closed fists, sneezing or retching, were generally used.

Convulsions were treated by bleeding, giving sneezing medicines and clysters, using emollients to dilate the cervix, blisters to the neck and arms, and plasters to the feet. It was generally agreed however that unless the woman could be speedily delivered she would almost certainly die. This accident, and severe haemorrhage before the delivery, were emergencies of such gravity that unless a fortunate termination occurred naturally, no midwife of the period — and only the best men-midwives — could have saved the woman, since the only possible recourse was immediate operative delivery.

Ante-partum haemorrhage, when not sudden and alarming, was often neglected, and the woman died. Willughby mentions three such cases: 'I knew three good women, the first flouded 1665, the second flouded 1666; The third flouded 1667. And this flux of blood continued, with some intermissions, for three, or foure weekes. These woman hoped, that the flux would have ceased of it self. But, through the oft returning, with the losse of much blood, they all (seeking for no help) died undelivered, none mistrusting any danger of death'.[22]

Haemorrhage after the birth, if severe, was generally fatal, since there was no effective method of arresting the flow, though several medicines and a cooling regimen were believed useful. Where the bleeding was caused by a retained placenta or fragments and clots, manual clearing of the womb might succeed, but midwives did not generally realise this, or know how to effect it. The treatment of post-partum haemorrhage was not only useless but positively pernicious, since it generally started with bleeding in the arm to make revulsion. Some women nevertheless recovered, which fostered the belief that the bleeding had done good. Portal reported such a case: 'I was called to a woman afflicted with a violent flux of blood, and who had evacuated a great quantity of coagulated blood before my coming. Considering she had strength enough as yet, I let her six ounces of blood, after which she fainted for half an hour, but then recovered. I conveyed my fingers into the neck of the womb, whence I brought forth many clods of coagulated blood. This, and a natural stool, gave her great ease, tho' the same is most to be attributed to the letting of blood, whereof I have had frequent experience in women troubled with the flux of blood'.[23]

Chapman on the other hand took a somewhat unorthodox line: 'In this Case I never Bleed, but lay the Patient very cool, almost naked, and cover her Body with Cloths dipped in *Water*, or *Vinegar* and *Water* mixed'.[24] Except for the novel rejection of bleeding, this method was an extension of the frequently advised cooling regimen, which involved laying skeins of wet silk in the groins, and cloths wet in vinegar and water to the loins, a method certainly known to, and used by, some midwives. Mauriceau however, having advised bleeding, clearing the womb manually, and the cold regimen, regretfully observed 'but if notwithstanding all this the Blood continues flooding, then the Woman will have often Fainting-fits, and be in great danger of losing her life; because one cannot apply in those places the Remedies fit for to stop the opening of the Vessels as we can in another'.[25]

Willughby doubted the worth of the usual medicines in really severe haemorrhage: 'where flouding issueth with a streame, I shall not easily bee perswaded, That filipendula roots, or succinum with yolkes of egges, or such like, will at all availe', though he used these remedies for want of better. In his view there was as yet no way to save a woman in such a case: 'I have known a few, that have recovered these fluxes; but I have heard of many, from midwives, and other women, that they have died of them. I hold the flux of blood deadly after delivery, if it bee great, I never heard of any woman, that escaped, but that they all perished'.[26]

*Chapter Twelve*

# 'The Manuall Practize' — Operative Delivery

It seems likely that in desperate cases surgeons had been called to save the life of a labouring woman by extracting the child with instruments long before *The birth of mankind* was published, although all the instruments then known were destructive and could not fetch a live child.

Despite the great faith placed in medicines *The birth of mankind* did include instructions to the midwife on how to deliver a dead child by hooks and knives, and also made reference to special surgical instruments for this purpose: 'But yf all these medicines profette not, then muste be used more seuere and harde remedyes, with instrumentes, as hokes, tonges, and suche other thynges made for the nonce . . . Yf it be so that it lye the head forewarde, then fasten a hoke other upo*n* one of the eyes of it, or the rofe of the mouthe, or under the chyn . . . and when this hoke is thus fastened . . . lette her [midwife] with her ryghte hande fasten another in some other parte of the byrthe ryght ageynste the fyrste' and so draw it out evenly. If a limb appeared and could not be reduced the midwife was told to cut it off, 'for the which purpose the surgeo*ns* haue mete instrumentes made for the nonce with the which such legges and armes may sone be cut frome the bodye'. If the head was swollen, 'that it wyl not conueneiently yssue oute that narowe places, then let the mydwyfe with a sharpe penknyfe cutte open the heade, that the humours contayned in it may yssue and runne forth'; but if the head was merely large rather than hydropical, 'then muste the head be broken in peces', and if necessary the body also.[1]

There were more complicated and specialised instruments, which were fully described and illustrated in Rueff's book, including the drake's bill, speculum, apertorium, and long tongs. All these were used as dilating instruments, and all except the speculum could also be used in the extraction of a dead birth. The gryphon's talon was specially designed to take hold of a round mass, and was used for extracting moles and the separated foetal head. Although Rueff's instructions were addressed to the midwife it is evident that she would be unlikely to possess these specialised instruments, and that where a case necessitated their use it would be the surgeon who brought them and used them.[2] As Rueff observed in his instructions, 'after the same manner we our selves have also oftentimes proceeded in these accidents and chances'.

It would be wrong to suppose that midwives did not operate however; Willughby mentioned several cases where they had done so, usually with ordinary household utensils such as hooked ladles, knives and needles, and usually with bad results. One such midwife asked permission to watch Willughby operate, and although he let her stand by she saw nothing, and he expressed himself 'willing to keep her in sufficient ignorance . . . not to encourage her in her evil wayes of using pothooks, or pot ladles, with which shee, formerly, had made ill work'. Another had tried for four days to deliver her patient by pulling on the child's scalp with threaded packneedles , 'but the skin was rotten, and quickly torn, and her hopes frustrated'. Yet another dismembered the child with a knife; 'Her knife, in doing this work, was broken with many great notches, as shee hackled in her body'. Willughby was shown the knife after the patient's death by the relatives, 'And all of them reviled this ignorant woman, and too late distasted her evil doings'.

He was of the opinion that midwives would be better advised to learn the use of the crochet, which was the instrument a surgeon would use, and that this was better done by watching a good surgeon operate than by reading books: 'But, if high, and lofty conceited midwives, that will leave nothing unattempted, to save their credits, and to cloak their ignorances, let mee advice such women to learn how to make use of the crochet, rather then pothooks, packneedles, silver spoones, thatcher's hooks, and knives, to shew their imagined skils. I have known the midwives, and the places, where they have used these follies to their women'.[3] Not many surgeons however would have been willing to instruct a midwife in the use of the crochet, and such instruction was without doubt easier wished for than obtained.

McMath did not illustrate any instruments, which he thought 'may, and ought, to be abandoned, for their pernicious Effects upon both Women and Children', though he was very vague about possible alternatives. Hugh Chamberlen, in his preface to Mauriceau, partly by way of advertising the family secret — the forceps — condemned the use of hooks by surgeons unless necessitated by some monstrous birth, and considered their use by midwives to be even more reprehensible, though some English midwives did use them, 'which rash presumption, in *France*, would call them in question for their lives'.[4]

However by the end of the seventeenth century it was generally accepted that if operative delivery was necessary, a man-midwife should be called in. Sermon, pointing out that if medicines failed instruments would be necessary, declined to go into detail, 'seeing such remedies are most commonly made use of by men, called to women in such a deplorable state, I shall here omit to make any farther mention of them'.[5]

Surgeons themselves sometimes had to use improvised instruments; Portal used the hook of an iron ladle struck into an eye socket in a case where the mother was in convulsions and he had no instruments with him, and also in another case when the husband refused to let him go home and fetch them for fear he would not return.

The crochet was a somewhat controversial instrument, partly because it could be dangerous for the mother and partly because it was sometimes used in error or on purpose on living children, who died as a result. Willughby said, 'I know not a better instrument, than the crochet, to help a woman in extremity, when shee is overwearied, and that her strength, with all other meanes, doth faile, and the woman's body very narrow, or strait, or swel'd by violent enforcements, and the child dead. But, if it bee not used with great care, and judgment, it may prove destructive, by ill fixing, as well as by tearing, and losing the hold, as also by hasty, and rash drawing, and so wound the woman'.

Willughby had reason to know some surgeons were not as expert as they should have been with the instrument: 'A Gentlewomen, and one nearly related to mee, was delivered by a man midwife, whilest that I dwelt at London . . . His instrument, as hee worked, did overslip his hand, and was heard to fall into the bason, and, in probability, the woman's body was wounded by his instrument, through his ill using of it. If this narration was truly related to mee, by those women, that were present at her delivery, his work was carried on with much unhandsomenes, and accompanied with great ignorance. Shee soon after rotted in the womb, from whence noisome vapors, and ill sented fluxes issued; and so this poor soul, within a few dayes after, miserably finished her life'.[6]

Some surgeons refused to operate if the woman seemed far spent, for fear of scandal: 'If every circumstance perswades, that the Operation would be in vain, 'tis better to let it alone, than she should dye under his hand, and he be blamed for it, and incur the name of Butcher, as is most certain when such a misfortune happens'.[7] But Read felt despite this risk ' 'tis better to attempt an operation of an incertain consequence, than to abandon the sick to certain despair; for sometimes Nature recovers beyond Hope'.[8]

If the crochet was attended with risk for the mother it was certainly fatal for the child, if not already dead, and there was much debate whether its use where the child was yet alive could be justified. The general weight of opinion was that since, where the birth was impossibly obstructed the child would die eventually, it was justifiable to use the crochet sooner, while the mother had strength to endure the operation, rather than later, when the fruitless labour had weakened her dangerously. But such a situation required much circumspection, and Willughby warned the midwife not to 'bee too hasty to send for a young chirurgeon, to extract the infant, and let her never put him forward to bee busy in such works . . . and, as long as the child is living, to have a tender conscience, not to destroy life, although it come in no good posture, but rather endeavour to amend the birth by their own practice, or by the help of others'.[9]

Unfortunately, it was very difficult to be certain foetal death had occurred until such signs as manifestly putrid discharges and odours, and a state of extreme deterioration in the mother, supervened, and at that late stage an operation would not necessarily save her. Additional and more reliable signs of foetal death, not noted earlier, were mentioned in the seventeenth century. If the fontanelle was soft and pulseless for example, or the cord prolapsed and ceased pulsation, the child was dead. Midwives tested where an arm or foot presented by dipping the part in cold water, believing that if the child was alive it would draw it in; but Read pointed out the unreliability of this sign, since the infant was often wedged so tightly that he could not draw back the protruding limb. It used to be said that the child was dead if meconium was passed, but this sign also came to be seen as unreliable; some surgeons found nothing more common in malpresentations, even where a live infant was born.[10]

Mauriceau, in advising that a prolapsed arm could be twisted off rather than cut, with less risk to the mother, emphasised that the surgeon must be very sure that the child was dead, 'for what a horrible spectacle would it be, to bring (as some have sometimes done) a poor Child yet living, after the Arm hath been cut off'.[11]

Guillemeau considered it permissible to use the crochet on a live child if the mother would certainly die otherwise, 'But I thinke, there are none, that goe about this businesse, but with some touch of Conscience'.[12] Willughby more than once consulted ministers of religion on the matter. In one case of severe ante-partum haemorrhage 'being unwilling to use any violence, I objected, what if the child should bee alive? Her husband prayed mee to use any meanes to save his wife's life, and a Priest, standing by him, willed mee, whether the child should bee living, or dead, to proceed, not valuing the child's life, saying, That, without all doubt, the child already was, or shortly would bee a Saint in heaven'.[13] This child was in fact dead, but on another occasion when the same advice was given he drew a live child with the crochet, which lived long enough to be immediately baptised.

Such cases not unnaturally made women put off calling a man-midwife, and often when he had behaved with the utmost circumspection a crochet delivery did his reputation no good. As Read advised, 'Althô the Chirurgeon be sure that the Child is dead in the Womb, and that it is necessary to fetch it by Art, he must not therefore presently use his Crotchets, because they are never to be used but when Hands are not sufficient . . . because, very often, thô he has done all that Art directs, persons present, that understand not these things, will believe that the Child was killed with the Crotchets, althô it had been dead three days before, and without other reasonings or better understanding of the matter, for recompence of his saving the Mother's life, requite him with an accusation, of which he is altogether innocent; and in case the Mother by misfortune should afterwards dye, lay her death also to his charge'.[14]

In many cases, often because the patient, her relatives, or the midwife resisted sending for a man-midwife, he was called in so late that the woman was almost moribund, and then he had the unenviable choice of attempting an operation with but the faintest chance of success, and leaving the patient to certain death. Mauriceau's own sister died in childbirth largely because a famous surgeon was afraid that if she died under his hands it would spoil his reputation with ladies of quality.

The opposite dilemma faced a surgeon where the woman seemed at death's door, but the child was probably alive. Caesarean section had been done post-mortem in ancient times, and was described in *The birth of mankind*. But in the second half of the sixteenth century it was proposed as a feasible operation on the living woman. The first such operation was done in 1500, reputedly successfuly, by a Swiss sow-gelder on his own wife.[15] Mercurio suggested it in cases of contracted pelvis in *La commare o riccoglitrice*, published in 1596, one of the first works to relate pelvic deformity to difficult labour. In 1581 Rousset enthusiastically recommended it, supporting his theoretical arguments with cases described to him by 'personnages non suspects'.[16]

Before this however Paré had already authorised the operation at the Hôtel Dieu on five occasions, as his pupil Guillemeau reported: 'Some hold, that this Cæsarian Section, may and ought to be practized (the woman being aliue) in a painfull and troublesome birth: Which for mine owne part, I will not counsell any one to do, hauing twise made triall of it my selfe, in the presence of *Mons. Paræus*, and likewise seen it done by *Mons. Viart*, *Brunet*, and *Charnonnet*, all excellent Chirurgeons, and men of great experience and practize; who omitted nothing, to doe it artificially, and methodically: Neuerthelesse, of fiue women, in whom this has been practized, not one hath escaped . . . After *Mons. Paræus* had caused vs to make triall of it, and seen that the successe was verie lamentable, and vnfortunate: he left of, and disallowed this kind of practize, together with the whole Colledge of Chirurgeons of Paris'.[17] Paré accordingly declared the operation impossible 'without the death of the mother . . . for the wombe of a woman that is great with childe . . . must needs yeeld a great flux of blood, which of necessity must be mortall . . . For these and such like other causes, this kinde of cure, as desperate and dangerous, is not (in mine opinion) to be used'.[18]

Mauriceau, in answer to the argument that women sometimes recover beyond expectation after caesarean section, declared 'I do utterly deny it, by the testimony of the most expert Chirurgeons that have practised it, who alwaies had bad success'. He continued, 'As for Paré, he will not acknowledg that he saw those two Operations of *Guillemeau*, because he will not have Posterity know that he was able to consent to so great a cruelty'.[19]

Willughby considered the operation theoretically possible: 'It is a work not difficult to performe. It hath been performed by ignorant men, and the women have recovered', but he nevertheless would not countenance it, 'For the Cæsarean Section, I do not like it'.[20]

It was not, indeed, a difficult operation, since the technique involved merely cutting into the uterus along a previously marked line, removing the child and placenta, and stitching up the abdomen. The uterus itself was not sutured, and many practitioners justly feared the resulting haemorrhage, but Rousset blithely stated it was not greater than in many normal births, and was only retained menstrual blood anyway.[21]

Evidently it was popularly believed that the operation could be, and had been, successfully done: 'There are many good Women who, for having only heard some Gossips speak of it, are very confident that they know such and such yet living, whose sides had been so opened to fetch the Child so out of their Belly'.[22] Barret also said 'Some Country Gossips will tell you they know such yet living, whose Sides have been opened to make way for the Child: But such Stories as these, are only fit Entertainment for Fools and Children'. Post-mortem caesarean section was however sometimes done.

Rousset had argued that the operation might be permissible for pressing political reasons, as did Pechey, 'when a Family is like to be extinguished; or some Kingdom or Principality is like to be lost'. But Mauriceau thought such a suggestion totally unethical. Despite the attention authors paid to the subject no successful caesarean section on a living woman was recorded in England until 1793.[23]

Even post-mortem caesarean section seems to have been quite unusual, though common enough in Catholic countries where the baptism of the child was considered more important. Read directed the incision to be made vertically through the rectus muscle, but other surgeons thought a semi-circular incision on the side of the abdomen was less likely to injure the child. Although by the late seventeenth century it was well known that the child's respiration depended on the mother, Sharp nevertheless claimed that the idea that the operation was pointless unless done immediately was 'an error, for the child hath a Soul and life of its own, and may live a while without the Mother; but the Midwife must keep the womb open that it be not stifled till the Chirurgeon cuts it out'.[24] Van Roonhuyse, arriving to do a post-mortem caesarean section, 'found the poor woman dead, having a key betwixt her teeth to keep her mouth open; which is practised among the vulgar, who thereby think for a while to keep the child alive'.[25]

At the time *The birth of mankind* was published, Paré and other surgeons in France were experimenting with the method of delivery by podalic version. This operation involved turning the child to the feet and drawing it out by traction on the legs, and in many cases offered an escape route from the difficult ethical dilemmas posed by the crochet and caesarean section. Its great advantage was that it could be used much sooner than either of the other two methods, thus offering some likelihood of the child being still alive, and the mother having strength enough to withstand the not inconsiderable shock and strain of the operation. Paré himself learned the technique from the successful practice of Thierry Hery and Nicole Lambert — master barber-surgeons in Paris — and published his directions in 1549. Until 1612 however, when Guillemeau's book was translated into English, instruction in the method was not available in any language a midwife could be expected to read. Many midwives indeed could not read at all, and were obliged to gain all their knowledge by hearsay and example.

Paré's own complete works were translated in 1634, and Harvey's work describing and advising podalic version appeared in English in 1653. But Paré's book is in a large format and very long, and was no doubt fairly expensive, and Harvey's is disguised by its title, so that it is unlikely that even the few literate midwives would be familiar with these books. The more popularly-written midwiferies however, such as Culpeper, Sharp and Sermon, made no mention of the technique. Not surprisingly therefore midwives carried on with the traditional methods, and by the end of the seventeenth century it had become an accepted fact that men-midwives were necessary in difficult cases, and that the best way a midwife could demonstrate her ability was in recognising complications promptly enough to call a man-midwife in good time.

There were no training courses in midwifery until the eighteenth century for either sex, but the better surgeons served proper apprenticeships, and had better access to books, and in London at least to anatomical teaching. During their apprenticeships they would be shown how to use instruments, and if apprenticed to a man-midwife who used the technique, how to do version.

The low general level of midwives' capacities is not surprising in view of the structure of society. Educated ladies and gentlewomen very rarely became professional midwives, though a few, such as Willughby's own daughter, did so.[26] She was taught to use podalic version successfully by him, but he seems never to have met with any other midwife who had even attempted the maneouvre, and the ordinary midwives to whom he taught it either forgot it or preferred their own methods. He showed a midwife how to manage a breech presentation in 1632, but when he was called to such another birth some years later attended by the same midwife, 'shee had forgotten what I shewed her, with all the directions. After twelve houres suffering under two midwives, this woman's friends perswaded her to send for mee, to assist, and help her, and her midwives. After I had seen the birth, I asked the midwife, if that, formerly, I had not shewed her this birth, and the way how to help it. At last shee remembered it'.[27] In another case a woman he had formerly laid by podalic version died in a subsequent birth after several midwives had pulled the child away from her by main force: 'Two of these midwives did formerly see mee lay these births by the feet. But midwives will follow their own wayes, and will have their own wills'.[28]

Many midwives were still following the advice of *The birth of mankind* and its popular successors to turn all malpresentations to the head. But Read commented that 'Some Authors who have written of Labours, and never practised them, do order all by the same precept often reiterated, that is, to reduce all wrong Births to a natural Figure; which is, to turn it, that it may come with the Head first: But if they themselves had ever had the least experience, they would know that it is very often impossible', and further even if accomplished, 'usually the Woman has no more Throws nor Pains fit for Labour, after she has been so wrought upon', whereas in a delivery by the feet they are not so essential.[29]

Willughby also emphasised the impossibility of dealing with unnatural births by turning to the vertex. But even where the child was dead, podalic version could be a useful procedure: 'where there is room to put up the hand . . . a woman may easier, and better bee delivered by the hand, and more sooner, then shee can bee by the crochet . . . And it will bee more pleasing to the woman to bee laid by the hand. For instruments bee dreadfull to them'.[30] On the other hand, he agreed with Guillemeau that when the child was dead and 'the child's head is much entered within the os pubis, it is impossible to thrust him upward to turn him, without much endangering the mother, and causing great contusion in the womb, from whence proceed diverse accidents, and sometimes death with them'.[31]

But whether the woman were to be delivered by version or the crochet, in either case it was usually necessary to send for a man-midwife, and authors repeatedly emphasised that it should be done in good time, and that women should commend midwives prepared to do this, rather than complain of their incapacity. As Chamberlen put it: 'Let me therefore advise good Women, not to be too ready to blame those Midwives skill, who are not backward in dangerous cases to desire advice; lest it cost them dear by discouraging them, and forcing them to presume beyond their knowledge, or strength especially, there being already but too-too-many over confident'.[32]

At some time in the seventeenth century the obstetric forceps were invented by a member of the Chamberlen family, thus enabling a difficult head presentation to be managed without version or the crochet. They were kept a family secret for about a century,[33] but were evidently in use, by some city men-midwives at least, before the first books describing their use were written. The first dated case in which Giffard used forceps was at a birth he attended in 1726, but his book was not published until 1734, the year after his death. In it appeared an illustration of his own forceps, and a version by another surgeon. In the previous year however an illustration of midwifery forceps had been presented to Edinburgh Medical Society by Alexander Butter. Nevertheless Chapman complained that using the crochet on a live and normally-presenting infant was still the custom of some 'rash, pretending, Artists'. He also said hooks were still used in such cases, 'a most cruel and unwarrantable Practice. But yet, however inhuman, it is, to my certain Knowledge, by Some kept up to this Day'.[34] However it was not long before every man-midwife had provided himself with the wonderful new instrument, or its relatives — the vectis and the lever — and the stage was set for the ferocious arguments of the eighteenth century over the unnecessary use of them.

*Chapter Thirteen*

# Two Centuries of Obstetric Change Reviewed

Beginnings are usually easier to establish than endings; we can say when a technique was first invented or a theory first propounded with much more certainty than we can assess how widely and quickly its influence was felt, or when it fell out of use or ceased to be accepted.

Historians of obstetrics, concentrating on great men and their discoveries, have sometimes painted a picture of progress from one milestone to another, forward to enlightenment, which does no sort of justice to the complexities of reality. Not only was such innovation not always an unqualified improvement, but it took place often in a context of resistance to new ideas, and always alongside the persistence of older ones. The desuetude of these older ideas is much harder to establish, not least because they made their last stand in the minds of uneducated women, a section of the population markedly unlikely to leave documentary record of its views.

Historians such as Aveling and Spencer in their anxiety to give credit where credit was due have also tended to minimise and underestimate the role of the patient in obstetric development. It must never be forgotten that obstetrics in our period was totally uninstitutionalised in this country. It was a paid personal service, except at the very lowest charity level, and the preferences, ideas and prejudices of the patient and other influential women about her, had much bearing on what a midwife or man-midwife could in practice do, since ultimately the obstetric attendant would be engaged again or not, recommended to friends or not, by these women. Therefore erroneous ideas held by the patient were often tactfully complied with; among many examples we may note holding the mouth and genitals of a dead woman open if post-mortem caesarean section was contemplated, disposing of the placenta by some means other than burning, and applying customary topics to repel the milk.

But the dynamics of this consumer situation did not always work in the patient's best interests; both men and women midwives seem often to have been under great pressure to take active measures even against their better judgement, for fear they should be thought ignorant or idle by the patient and her friends. Similarly many medicines continued to be given and practices maintained long after they were considered useless on scientific grounds, merely to satisfy the patient. In other cases it may have proved impossible to apply new techniques or to undertake necessary procedures, especially where these were likely to be painful, because the patient refused consent.

Men-midwives, perhaps partly because they knew there was a strong initial prejudice against them to be overcome on account of their sex, seem to have been more aware of the necessity of conciliating the patient than midwives, some of whom adopted a bossy and domineering manner. The sort of midwife who reproved a woman frightened and in pain with a sharp reminder that she herself had had ten children with no such fuss could not in the nature of things have a male counterpart. It may be suspected that the greater diplomacy of men-midwives, quite as much as their superior strength and technical expertise, in some measure contributed to a success in encroaching on the midwives' traditional domain that certainly calls for explanation.

In attempting to assess what changes actually came about in women's beliefs and practices in this period, as distinct from changes described in books, it must be freely admitted that lack of documentation makes such assessments a speculative business, and conclusions about them necessarily tentative and provisional.

We simply do not know how far women relied on common sense and personal experience, how far they were influenced by traditional women's lore, nor how widely read and influential the better books were. In some respects working-class women may have 'known' more than the better educated and their professional attendants. It seems quite credible that they knew from practical experience that lactation had a contraceptive effect, that the longer the pregnancy continued the likelier the child was to survive, that nine months was the normal length of gestation, that colostrum did the baby no harm, nor did coitus during nursing, that menstruation did not depend on the phases of the moon, and that menstrual blood was not poisonous. But it is at least equally credible that they accepted the erroneous but ancient views expressed in contemporary popular literature. Certainly the contents of the *Aristotle* books suggest that many notions long abandoned by the educated were still very much alive at a popular level.

Some ideas current at the start of our period were however almost certainly obsolete by 1750; that the uterus had seven cells for example, that the female genitals were the same as the male reversed, that witchcraft could cause sterility, that amulets or tossing the woman in a blanket would help obstructed labour. But many more ideas denounced as erroneous in the books quite certainly persisted; superstitions about the caul,[1] belief in uroscopy, beliefs about 'longings' and birthmarks, that female orgasm was necessary for conception,[2] or that hysteria was caused by vapours.

Many of these ideas did no great harm, but ignorance of anatomy and physiology on the other hand often had unfortunate practical consequences. Midwives who imagined a child could stick to the mother's back were tempted to interfere internally in an effort to free it.[3] They did not understand the structure of the pelvis, and thought protruding arms and legs could be used to pull the child out. Similar ignorance prevented them from realising that a malformed pelvis or a protruding coccyx could not be overcome by stretching the vagina and a dose of the midwife's powder. Most midwives made vaginal examinations, but some could not even tell what stage labour had reached by this means. Very few could deal with an arm presentation or a retained placenta, and emergencies such as placenta praevia were quite beyond their understanding. A similar lack of technical expertise was also found in some men-midwives, but the best were without doubt superior to the best women in abnormal cases, and therefore began to be employed in preference to them for the sake of safety by women of means.

Wealthier women therefore probably fared better in emergencies and difficulties than those who could not afford a man-midwife, or lived in areas remote from such help. In normal births however their midwives may have been more inclined to show off their skills and to interfere unnecessarily in the birth than the midwives of the poor. Lying-in customs favoured by the rich furthermore were less healthy than those of the poor. Early rising out of bed, eating a normal diet and nursing one's own child must have produced better results than lying in a dark hot room for many days, living on liquids and repelling the milk with poultices. Indeed Willughby and others pointed out that those who had no attendants at all, vagrants for example, often had the easiest and healthiest births of all, and the best midwives in a normal birth were those who did least.

There was in this period a distinct movement from implicit acceptance of humoral medicine and medical methods of dealing with labour, especially in difficulties, towards reliance on manual and surgical means. Although faith in humoral medicine was declining in other areas of practice also, in obstetrics the process was particularly marked. It was a field in which the failure of humoral medicine was early and clearly demonstrated, and where manual and surgical expertise was plainly seen to have more therapeutic value than the prescriptions of the learned physician. It is indeed probable that some of the hostility later shown to men-midwives by other medical men arose from jealousy at their more obvious success, which gave the man-midwife what his rivals considered a mean advantage in securing general practice in families.

Improvements in obstetrics were effected in two ways, first by the discrediting and abandonment of ineffective methods, such as reliance on amulets and birth powders, rolling women on the bed or turning malpresentations to the vertex, and second by the introduction of new and more successful methods. These methods were devised in response to improved theoretical knowledge, and to informed observation in clinical practice, very often with both these elements reinforcing each other. The most important of these advances concerned the management of obstructed labour, and certain emergencies such as placenta praevia, post-partum haemorrhage and retained placenta.

Improved knowledge of anatomy soon made it obvious that an infant presenting in certain postures could not emerge through the pelvis without correcting the position. As the structure of the normal pelvis became better understood it was also realised that abnormalities such as a narrow or deformed outlet or an inwardly-projecting coccyx also caused obstructed labour. Men-midwives found that in many cases podalic version provided a more ethically acceptable solution than the former expedient of crochet delivery, and a more clinically-effective one than turning to the vertex. Because it allowed the operator not only to alter the position of the foetus, but by traction on the legs to supply the deficiencies in the mother's own expulsive powers, podalic version also enabled the operator to shorten labour where necessary in other difficulties such as uterine inertia, haemorrhage and convulsions.

A more exact understanding of the uterine action seems to have been rather the result of shrewd clinical deduction than of abstract theory. It was observed early that expulsive pains were useless until full dilation of the cervix had occurred, and good practitioners waited until they could ascertain by vaginal examination that this stage had been reached before urging the patient to bear down, although this point was perhaps less-widely understood than it should have been. When it was understood that the uterus expelled the child rather than the child forcing its own way out it was more evident that ineffective uterine action needed assistance by version, or later by the still better expedient of the forceps. Fumigations, birth powders and birth stones were then abandoned.

It also became clear that the uterus itself stopped bleeding from the placental site, and this had important practical implications. Placenta praevia could not be helped by the old method of replacing the detached placenta, indeed, even where the placenta was only partially detached the haemorrhage would continue until the uterus was emptied. Paré's advice to open the cervix manually or with instruments and deliver the woman immediately by podalic version was a real advance, although it needed a bold and knowledgeable operator, and was attended by risk of shock and sepsis.

It also followed that post-partum haemorrhage was caused by the uterus failing to contract, and men-midwives began to try clearing the womb manually to remove any obstacles to its contraction. Retained placenta was also dealt with by this method, rather than by the old combination of traction on the cord, expulsive medicines and suppurative injections. External manual expression was also in use, but failed to become universally adopted. Haemorrhage remained a dangerous complication, but manual clearing of the uterus must have helped in some of these cases, though again the risk of sepsis made its value less unequivocal than it seemed to contemporaries.

Better understanding of the circulation of the blood and the function of the placenta in supplying the place of breathing for the infant showed the importance of prompt delivery where the cord prolapsed or was compressed. For the same reason where the placenta was detached, delivery was as vital for the infant as for the mother. The prompt use of version or the forceps in such cases must have improved the prospects of survival for the infant.

There were unfortunately drawbacks to these new techniques, mainly the problem of sepsis, but the time was yet to come when the importance of hygiene would be discovered. The general trend towards needless interference in normal labour by 'haling' midwifery — so unfortunately promoted in the earlier part of the period — had been put into reverse by the end, and this too must count as an improvement.

During these two centuries midwifery passed from a female mystery employing traditional medicines and often superstitions, even in difficult cases, to a scientifically-based clinical skill, with both gains and losses to the patient. Some of the psychological satisfaction and social bonding of the old ways was sacrificed for the safety of the patient in difficult cases. In the process the status of the midwife was seriously threatened by the coming of the man-midwife.

The importance of men's new involvement in midwifery is very evident, whether as anatomists and physiologists discovering new facts, surgeons devising new techniques, the Chamberlens inventing the forceps, or authors bringing these matters to the attention of practitioners. Given the limited educational opportunities of women in general and midwives in particular, scientific enlightenment and technical improvement could have come no other way. And on balance if the female midwives lost by these changes, the patients gained. Opponents of men-midwives in the eighteenth century often presented them as exploiters of female ignorance and folly, but it seems more likely their success was due to a quite rational evaluation by women themselves of the respective merits of male and female midwives, and a conscious decision to employ men in defiance of sexual prejudice in the interests of the women's own safety and comfort.

*Appendix*

# Maternal Mortality: Some Notes on the Willughby Cases

It is clear from the evidence already adduced that a high maternal mortality rate could be expected in the sixteenth and seventeenth centuries. Indeed, although the ascendancy of the man-midwife and the popularisation of the forceps in the eighteenth century almost certainly reduced both the number of women dying undelivered, and the number of stillborn babies, it is possible that in a pre-aseptic era, post-partum maternal deaths from sepsis and puerperal fever may even have increased. By 1793 Blunt observed 'we seldom hear of a woman dying in labour, although many die in childbed'.[1]

Pilot studies suggest that the maternal mortality rate in the sixteenth and seventeeth centuries may have been as high as 25 per 1000 birth events, some five or six times higher than the official figures for the nineteenth century.[2] The Registrar-General was certainly right when in his 1857 report he claimed, 'Childbirth is much more fatal than it should be; but much less fatal than it was'.

Maternal mortality figures for the period before 1837, when civil registration of births and deaths was instituted, are not easy to obtain, and those obtained from parish registers by the conventional method of correlating burials of mothers with infant baptisms always err on the optimistic side because they omit two significant groups of maternal fatalities. These are women dying undelivered, and women dying in childbed of stillborn children.[3]

The cases reported by Willughby alone however make it clear that many mothers did die undelivered, and many others after difficult and tedious labours, often involving operative delivery, such as tended to end in the birth of a dead child.

Major causes of death undelivered, which, as we have already seen, the usual methods pursued by midwives were quite unable to deal with, must include ante-partum haemorrhage, convulsions, disproportion and pelvic deformity, difficult malpresentations, and uterine inertia. In virtually all of these cases spontaneous delivery, though possible, was not very likely.

The gravity of ante-partum haemorrhage was first realised by Paré, and it was to meet this particular emergency that he originally recommended podalic version, with manual dilation of the cervix if necessary. Willughby noted that neglect of this condition led to death undelivered. No less a person than Lady Lowther died in this way in 1648. According to her husband's diary she was 'then at hir accommpt of ye 12th [child] wherof it pleased God shee dyed not delivered . . . Shee had a great breach about 7 weekes before shee dyed which brough[t] hir weake yet shee recovered that and at ye 5 weekes end had another breach untill when shee felt ye [child] to stirr and ye issue of Blood Continued with hir [until] Wedenday night shee dyed; in which tyme shee was h[ourely] afflicted with extremitie of sicknesse and yett noe tra[vell] upon hir to deliv[er] the birth'.[4] It does not seem that any attempt was made to deliver Lady Lowther by version or by instruments, and it is unlikely many women of inferior social status would have had better care.

Where the placenta actually came out first, most men-midwives of the time would have attempted delivery, but where bleeding was the only symptom they, as well as the female midwives, may well have put off the operation until too late, either for fear of the effect on the patient of operative delivery, or less nobly, for fear of the effect on their credit if it failed.

Convulsions, whether epileptic or eclamptic, might also cause the death of the mother undelivered, as Willughby reported in the case of a young woman 'supposed to bee in labour of her first child . . . January the 29 at eight a clock at night shee fell into convulsion fits, and, without any intermission, continued in them untill past one the next day, and senseles died in them'.[5]

Disproportion between the child's head and the pelvis might also cause the mother to die undelivered: 'where the head and body bee too great, shee will not be delivered, nor the child saved, unles the birth bee turned from the head to the feet, and afterward to bee, by the feet, produced'.[6] Even in a tedious but otherwise normal labour where the mother's strength was failing she might be unable to give birth. In such a case terminated by podalic version Willughby said: 'Had I not drawn the child by the feet, the mother would not have been delivered. And, if that I still had deferred time, in hopes to have had a natural birth, this child, born so weak, would have perished in the mother's womb, and the mother with it, and they would not have been separated'.[7] It was this type of case especially which might be expected to become much rarer after the forceps came into general use.

Closely associated with this problem was pelvic deformity, often due to rickets. It has been noted that rickets and its attendant obstetric risk seems to have been rare in prehistoric times,[8] but by the seventeenth century, when large numbers of people were brought up in poor urban environments, dietary habits had changed, and tight corseting even of small children was the fashion, rickets had evidently become common.[9]

Few midwives could have delivered a woman with any appreciable degree of pelvic deformity. A patient who had previously been delivered by Willughby as an emergency, when the midwives could not effect it, died undelivered in a subsequent labour when he was away: 'the midwife told mee, That the child never descended, or came within the bones, and that her body being narrow, shee knew not how to deliver her; and that it was past her understanding; and these things I knew well enough'.[10]

In one rachitic case of this kind podalic version and instruments were both insufficient to deliver the patient. Willughby gives a long circumstantial account of his efforts to deliver this lady, who had 'the passages very narrow, ovally formed, and the bones not far distant the one from the other . . . I endeavoured to turn the birth . . . but could not possibly effect it, for that I could not slide up any part of my hand into her body'. Being pressed to use instruments, 'I was much unwilling to use these wayes, for I feared, by reason of the narrow passage of her body, that I could not do it', and indeed so it proved; 'I could not get up my hand over any part of the head, to fix the instrument . . . I, diverse times, altered the instrument, but all would not do any good. So I was necessitated to desist, without any hopes of delivery, not knowing which way to relieve her, and shee died'.[11]

Willughby claimed to have left only this one patient undelivered in 45 years of practice, but it is clear that many of the rachitic patients he delivered, except in the most expert hands, would have shared this lady's fate. Indeed, even after the forceps came into common use, such a patient would still have been impossible to deliver, since extreme pelvic contraction is one of the few absolute indications for caesarean section.[12]

Malpresentations, especially where they were mismanaged, were another cause of death undelivered. Many of the emergencies Willughby attended were malpresentations, especially impacted arm presentations, abandoned as hopeless by the midwives. Willughby blamed cutting the membranes too soon for some of these cases. The attempts of midwives to deal with the problem by reducing the arm and turning to the vertex were unlikely to succeed, but since they knew no better way such patients must often have died undelivered. And if a woman survived the actual delivery she was often so afflicted with shock, bruising and lacerations, that after the child had been pulled from her dead, she herself did not survive long.

Quoting the directions given in such cases by Sermon and Wolveridge, which did not include podalic version, Willughby observed, 'I could wish that these wayes, thus expressed by these worthies, might prove effectuall, and have an happy successe, the which, as yet, I could not, at any time, see to bee performed'. He considered the arm presentation the most frequently mismanaged by midwives: 'This is the birth, which most amazeth, and puzleth midwives, and bringeth into their thoughts unhandsome performances, so that . . . they become bold, with forcible halings, to pull off the armes, and shoulders of children into severall pieces in the mother's womb, to bring forth the body, thus killing the child, and, oft, the mother with it'.[13]

The reason why maternal deaths were more frequent after stillbirths is that the cause of the stillbirth was often a long, difficult delivery, at worst mismanaged, at best needing manual or instrumental intervention. Any birth which involved such interference in the birth canal was likely to prove ultimately fatal to the mother. Crochet delivery, even well performed, could end in death: 'Sometimes women, after long travailing, and no hopes of delivery left, being weake, and wearied with paine, not finding any comfort by medicine, or the midwife, at last have desired help by the extraction of the child by the crochet, the which they have cheerfully, and well endured. Yet, not long after the fetching of the after-burden, they have died; perhaps some, through flouding; others, through weaknes, or thinnes of blood, or putrefaction in the womb'.[14]

In other cases podalic version was followed by death, as with another rachitic patient: 'through the ill position of the bones, the child could not descend. Being desirous to save the child's life, I turned the child in the womb. Although I have known severall children born with more trouble, and greater extremity, and live; yet this child was dead before shee was delivered. And shee herself lived but a very short time after her delivery'.[15]

Often the exact cause of death in such cases is obscure, but may sometimes have been concealed internal haemorrhage: 'Some women, within an houre's space after delivery, will begin to complain that they bee not well. If this paine continue, and their countenances alter, growing wan, and dusky, and that they, every day, grow worser, and fainter, and that they seem mopish, and altered in their understandings, their recovery is to bee feared. This affliction followeth many women after hard labour, and chiefly those, which have received bruises, or hurts in utero, vel vaginâ uteri, and they live not past a week, and usually they die about that time'.[16]

Fainting fits may suggest the same cause, or possibly embolism: 'A Gentlewoman, at Quinborrow in Leicester-shire, had fainting fits in her labour. Shee was delivered of a dead child. Shee much fainted, when the after-birth by her ignorant, fumbling midwife was endeavoured to bee fetched. I was compelled to help her, for feare shee should have died under her hands. These fainting fits much weakened her spirits. Shee daily decayed by them, and, within the moneth of her lying in child-bed, shee died'.[17]

The diarrhoea Willughby described as fatal in other cases may have been connected with sepsis; 'Scouring for the most part proves fatall, if that it happen in the first seven dayes. And it is much to bee feared, although it come twelve, or fourteen dayes after delivery. I have known it fatall to severall women, yet some few have recovered'.[18]

Puerperal fever must certainly have been a common sequel to interference in the birth canal with unwashed hands and instruments. Willughby himself paid little attention to it, but his contemporary Willis declared it was 'a very dangerous Fever, with a horrible Apparatus of Symptoms', 'which, by reason of its Mortality, deserves to be call'd Malignant'.[19] Certainly in the nineteenth century, after the Registrar-General's reports began to divide maternal deaths by cause, puerperal fever accounted for over half the deaths.

The universal practice of fetching the placenta by the sixteenth century method of traction on the cord might well have produced shock and post-partum haemorrhage in some cases. The method which superseded it however, manual removal, was more likely to lead to inflammation and sepsis, especially if the uterus was scratched, or part of the placenta left behind: 'If any part of the after-burden bee left sticking to the uterus, the after-purgings will flow forth evil sented, greene, and as if they proceeded from a dead body, and, sometimes, the courage, and strength of the womb being quite vanquished, a sudden gangrene doth induce a certain death'.[20] Thus in another case 'A Husbandman's wife at Littleore, nigh Darby, was much disquieted with the midwife, whilest that shee searched to find the after-birth. It was not found, but remained in her body. Shee grew a little unruly, and altered in her complexion, which turned blackish. And although it came away, of itself, three, or foure dayes after her delivery, yet shee died, about the yeare, 1636'.[21]

If some maternal deaths were caused by failure to operate, some were certainly caused by operating badly. Both midwives and men-midwives were guilty of this, but midwives, although they operated less often, because of their inexperience, lack of anatomical knowledge and of proper instruments, probably had worse success. A midwife at Ticknall 'endeavoured, in the same towne, to deliver a potter's wife by quartering the skull with a knife, and taking forth the braines, yet shee could not bring forth the child. But shee much hurted the woman. Her ignorance, with the woman's afflictions, stopt her for proceeding any farther. So her husband came to mee. I went to her with him. I sent for the midwife, and drew the child with the crochet, as shee stood by mee . . . This poore woman died the next day, I beleeve, through the hurts, that shee received from her midwife's knife . . . At Spoondon in Darbyshire another midwife used the same practice, for cutting the child's head, and pulling out the braines. In her sufferings I was sent for, but this midwife had finished her work before I came. And her woman died the next day after her delivery'.[22]

A normal birth, which was no doubt then as now the most common, was no more, or not much more, dangerous in the sixteenth and seventeenth centuries than it is now, unless poor midwifery made it so. But the least complication carried a much higher risk, though just how high has yet to be established.

# Notes

## Chapter One English Obstetrical Textbooks Before 1740

1. E. Mason-Hohl, *The diseases of women by Trotula of Salerno. A translation of Passionibus muliebris curandorum* (Los Angeles, 1940) pp. 1–2.

2. E.g. parts of Mss Additional 34111, Sloane 121, Sloane 5, Royal 18 A VI, Sloane 421a, Sloane 2463, Bodley Douce 37 and Bodley 483. Sloane 2463 has recently been edited with a modern English translation: B. Rowland, *Medieval woman's guide to health* (Kent State University Press, Ohio and Croom Helm, London, 1981).

3. A. Eccles, 'The early use of English for midwiferies 1500–1700', *Neuphilologische Mitteilungen*, vol. 78, no. 4 (1977), pp. 377–85.

4. T. Raynald, *The birth of mankind* (1545) the prologue.

5. J. Ballantyne, 'The "Byrth of Mankynde" ' (London, 1907) reprinted from *Journ. Obs. & Gyn. Brit. Emp.*

6. The quotations in this book are taken from the 1755 edition in each case.

7. A technique, still occasionally used, of assisting obstructed labours by turning the child in the womb to present by the feet, so that traction can be applied to the legs.

8. J. Rueff, *The expert midwife* (1637) p. 48.

9. N. Culpeper, *A directory for midwives* (1651) p. 172.

10. C.R., *The compleat midwife's practice enlarged*, 2nd edn (1659) preface.

11. J. Hester, *Three exact pieces of Leonard Phioravant* (1657) a prefatory letter signed W.I.

12. Ms Sloane, 1954.

13. There were doubtless earlier versions of this, which contained 'Physicall experiments presented to our late Queen Elizabeth's own hands', and had very old-fashioned contents.

14. A. Eccles, 'The reading public, the medical profession, and the use of English for medical books in the 16th and 17th centuries' *Neuphilologische Mitteilungen*, vol. 75, no. 1 (1974) pp. 143–56.

15. This edition is not in the British Library; the quotations are taken from the 1763 edition.

## Chapter Two The Legacy of the Ancients, and William Harvey

1. There were in fact many new schools of thought and varieties of opinion, but the version of humoral medicine presented to the lay reader tended to give the impression that there were no such differences, and that it was a body of agreed factual knowledge.

2. C.E. Rosenberg, 'The medical profession, medical practice and the history of medicine' in E. Clarke (ed.), *Modern methods in the history of medicine* (Athlone Press, London, 1971) p. 30.

3. R. Turner, *De morbis foemineis: the woman's counsellour* (1686) pp. 41–2.

4. N. Fontanus, *The womans doctour* (1652) pp. 37–8.
5. M. La Vauguion, *A compleat body of chirurgical operations* (1699) p. 242.
6. T. Willis, *The London practice of physick* (1685) p. 630.
7. Issues were wounds deliberately made in order to allow the humours to discharge. They were kept open, frequently for long periods, by the insertion of a foreign body such as a seton of silk thread.
8. Culpeper, p. 102.
9. L. Riverius, *The practice of physick* (1655) p. 529.
10. J. Guillemeau, *Child-birth: or the happy deliverie of women* (1612) pp. 224–5. The use of bleeding in uterine haemorrhage, based on the mechanical theory of revulsion, seems to have been abandoned as therapy by the later-eighteenth century. Chapman however was the only author in this period who did not employ it. In fever on the other hand bleeding continued in use long afterwards, since other reasons were advanced in favour of it in such cases which were not only not contradicted by the circulation but even supported by it. Puerperal fever patients were still being bled to syncope in the nineteenth century, e.g. Marshall Hall, *Commentaries on some of the more important diseases of females* (1827) p. 189. There was indeed some opposition to bloodletting, especially by the Paracelsians, in the seventeenth century, but not because of Harvey's discovery of the circulation. See A.B. Davis, *Circulation physiology and the medical chemistry in England 1650–1680* (Coronado Press, Lawrence, Kansas, 1973).
11. Ms Sloane 421A f.5r–v.
12. e.g. J. Pechey, *The compleat midwife's practice enlarged* 5th edn (1698) pp. 264–5. Referred to henceforth as Pechey II.
13. J. Wolveridge, *Speculum matricis* (1671) p. 10.
14. J. Sharp, *The midwives book* (1671) pp. 6–7.
15. N. Sudell, *Mulierum amicus* (1666) p. 7.
16. C.R., p. 222.
17. Sharp, pp. 12–13.
18. Rueff, p. 32.
19. F. Mauriceau, *The diseases of women with child and in child-bed*, tr. Hugh Chamberlen (1683) p. 20. Referred to henceforth as Mauriceau II.
20. F. Mauriceau, *The accomplisht midwife*, tr. Hugh Chamberlen (1673) p. 85. Referred to henceforth as Mauriceau I.
21. Pechey II, p. 3.
22. The change in colour of the blood in the lungs during pulmonary circuit was noted by Columbus in the mid-sixteenth century and widely accepted thereafter, but not by Harvey. Most of those who accepted this change did not however connect it with the absorption of any material substance from the air. A long line of authors from Paracelsus to Mayow accepted that the blood in the lungs absorbed some kind of 'nitro-aerial' particles from the air, but many of these theorists did not subscribe to Columbus' ideas about pulmonary transit, though many did believe in some kind of 'circulation' of blood. Mayow's originality lay in providing in 1677 elegant experimental demonstration for the nitro-aerial particles, which he and his contemporaries (Boyle for example) believed were important for sustaining life. But this was not really the same as Lavoisier's 'oxygen' theory, which was essentially new.
23. W. Harvey, *Anatomical exercitations, concerning the generation of living creatures. To which are added, particular discourses of births, and of conceptions etc.* (1653) p. 482. See R.G. Frank jr., *Harvey and the Oxford physiologists: a study of scientific ideas* (U. California Press Berkeley, LA, 1980) pp. 221–78.
24. A. Read: *Chirurgorum comes* (1687) pp. 582–3.

## Chapter Three The Legacy of the Ancients, and the Anatomists

1. C.D. O'Malley, *Andreas Vesalius of Brussels 1514–1564* (U. California Press,

Berkeley, LA, 1964) p. 56.

2. Ibid., p. 50.

3. L. di Capoa, *The uncertainty of the art of physick* (1684) p. 94.

4. Culpeper, p. 5.

5. W. Harvey, *The anatomical exercises . . . of 1653*, ed. G, Keynes (Nonesuch Press, London, 1928) editor's note.

6. E. Gasking, *Investigations into generation 1651–1828* (Hutchinson, London, 1967) p. 32.

7. Richard Kay saw such an exhibition from London, accompanied by lectures, first at Manchester and some months later at Bury, in 1742. W. Brockbank and F. Kenworthy (eds.), *The diary of Richard Kay a Lancashire doctor 1716–51* (Chetham Society XVI Third series, Manchester, 1968) p. 52. The techniques of preserving specimens in alcohol and by wax injection were both developed in the seventeenth century, and by 1700 substantial permanent collections existed in several places. The collection at the Anatomy school in Oxford, which was visited by Evelyn and his wife in 1650 had been greatly developed by 1681, when Charles II inspected it. H.M. Sinclair and A.H.T. Robb-Smith, *A short history of anatomical teaching in Oxford* (OUP, Oxford, 1950) p. 14.

8. P. Willughby, *Observations in midwifery* (SR publishers, Wakefield, 1972) p. 254. Because of this popular abhorrence the legislature were able to use dissection after execution as a mark of obloquy, as an alternative to hanging in chains.

9. Mauriceau I, p. 281.

10. Sharp, p. 133; Culpeper, p. 55.

11. F. Glisson, *A treatise of the rickets* (1651) pp. 9–10.

12. W. Giffard, *Cases in midwifery* (1734) Case 137 p. 380.

## Chapter Four The Female reproductive System

1. *Dr. Chamberlain's midwives practice* (1668) p. 25.

2. J. McMath, *The expert midwife* (1694) p. 11.

3. T. Johnson (tr.), *The workes . . . of Ambroise Paré* (1634) p. 947.

4. H. Crooke, *Mikrocosmographia*, 2nd edn (1631) p. 307.

5. Paré, p. 128.

6. N. Culpeper and A. Cole (trs.), *Bartholinus anatomy* (1668) p. 62.

7. J.Pechey, *A general treatise of the diseases of maids, big-bellied women, child-bed women, and widows* (1696) p. 57. Henceforth referred to as Pechey I.

8. O'Malley, p. 32.

9. W.L.H. Duckworth (tr.), *Galen on anatomical procedures: the later books* (Duckworth, Cambridge, 1962) pp. 112–13.

10. Raynald, f.13r.

11. Sharp, pp. 38–9.

12. Guillemeau, p. 236.

13. Dr Chamberlain, pp. 57–9.

14. Sharp, p. 79.

15. Ibid., p. 38.

16. Guillemeau, pp. 107–8.

17. Sharp, p. 53.

18. O'Malley, p. 95.

19. Mauriceau I, p. 283.

20. E. Chapman, *A treatise on the improvement of midwifery*, 2nd edn (1735), p. 152.

21. Mauriceau I, p. 258.
22. The spots on the uterus drawing from da Carpi represent these cotyledons.
23. O'Malley, p. 174. In the 1543 *Fabrica* this point was not made.
24. R. Barret, *A companion for midwives, childbearing women, and nurses* (1699) pp. 48–9.
25. P. Dionis, *A general treatise of midwifery* (1719) p. 31.
26. Rueff, p. 52.
27. Riverius, p. 422.
28. G. Fallopius, *Opera* (1600) p. 438
29. O'Malley, p. 144.
30. Pechey II, p. 36.
31. Ibid., p. 46.
32. Ibid., p. 42.
33. Gasking, p. 37.
34. Dr Chamberlain, p. 28.
35. Riverius, p. 422.
36. Mauriceau I, pp. 12–13.
37. Pechey II, pp. 43–4. Elsewhere however Pechey continued to write as if women did have seed. Many authors' writings demonstrate that although they were aware of, and assented to, the latest theories, they did not really integrate them into their thought system to the exclusion of old errors.

## Chapter Five Sexuality and Conception

1. N. de Venette, *The mysteries of conjugal love reveal'd* 3rd edn (1712) p. 22.
2. McMath, pp. 21–2.
3. Sharp, p. 45.
4. Dionis, p. 40.
5. J. Maubray, *The female physician* (1730) p. 378.
6. Pechey I, p. 54.
7. Pechey II, p. 37.
8. S. Edwards, *Female sexuality and the law* (Martin Robertson and Co., London, 1981) pp. 123–5.
9. Dionis, p. 64.
10. *Aristotle's experienced midwife* (1755) pp. 20–21. Henceforth referred to as Aristotle II. In their modern studies Masters and Johnson have reported a number of women interpreting orgasm subjectively as a sensation of emission. W.H. Masters and V.E. Johnson, *Human sexual response* (Churchill, London, 1966) p. 135.
11. P. Barrough, *The methode of physick* (1583) p. 157.
12. Sharp, p. 22.
13. Pechey II, p. 21.
14. J. Sadler, *The sicke womans private looking-glass* (1636) pp. 118–19.
15. C.R., p. 288.
16. Dr Chamberlain, p. 9.
17. Bartholin, p. 55.
18. Mauriceau I, pp. 45–6.
19. These theories, which have been well described by Gasking and also in J. Needham, *A history of embryology* 2nd edn (CUP, Cambridge, 1969), were known to the non-academic public only in the simplified forms incorporated in the popular textbooks. Harvey's work was however translated into English two years after its publication, and was therefore theoretically available to the public directly, unlike the work of other eminent embryologists.
20. Bartholin, p. 69–70.
21. Mauriceau I, p. 7.

22. Ibid., pp. 27–8.
23. Crooke, pp. 280–2.
24. Pechey II, p. 7.
25. Bartholin, p. 68.
26. N. Highmore, *The history of generation* (1651) p. 31.
27. McMath, p. 14.
28. Ibid., p. 40.
29. Mauriceau I, p. 45.
30. Ibid., pp. 47–8.
31. McMath, pp. 42–3.
32. Mauriceau I, pp. 52–3. Willughby made the same observation pp. 48–9.
33. Wiltshire Record Office $79^{B}/36$ p. 12.
34. Harvey, pp. 539–47.
35. Dionis, pp. 79–80.
36. Pechey I, p. 56. In his second book he supported the ovum theory less guardedly, but had by no means abandoned the two seeds theory.
37. Pechey II, p. 47.
38. Dionis, p. 59.
39. *Aristotle's masterpiece* (1755) p. 20. Henceforth referred to as Aristotle I.

## Chapter Six Development and Birth of the Foetus

1. The terms actually used were 'veiny artery' and 'still vein'. Much confusion and difficulty of interpretation is caused in these texts not only by the fluid state of the concepts, but by the even more fluid state of the vocabulary, now struggling to find English translations for the original Latin of the research work. See A. Eccles, 'The use of English for treatises on obstetrics from the 15th century to 1700', unpublished PhD thesis, University of London, 1974.
2. K.D. Keele, *William Harvey* (Nelson, London, 1965) p. 184.
3. Paré, p. 888.
4. McMath, p. 112.
5. Maubray, p. 30. Just one year before Maubray wrote this it had been experimentally disproved, Needham, p. 58.
6. Harvey, pp. 477–8.
7. McMath, p. 36.
8. 10 and 11 William III Cap.16.
9. J.T. Noonan, *The morality of abortion* (Harvard UP Cambridge, Mass., 1970) p. 27.
10. Read, pp. 538–9.
11. Paré, pp. 901–2.
12. Maubray, pp. 140–1.
13. Mauriceau I, p. 50.
14. Ibid., pp. 15–16.
15. Sharp, p. 122.
16. J. Leake, *A lecture introductory to the theory and practice of midwifery*, 3rd edn (1773) p. 25.
17. Raynald, f.45r.
18. The two illustrations are reproduced in O'Malley, Plate 53.
19. Paré, p. 133.
20. Mauriceau I, pp. 151–2.
21. Pechey II, p. 97.
22. Sharp, p. 143.
23. Raynald, f.44v–45r.
24. Wiltshire Record Office $79^{B}/36$ p. 3v.

25. J. Freind, *Emmenologia* (1703) pp. 1–8. An English translation of this work by T. Dale appeared in 1729.
26. The capillaries had been discovered by Malpighi in 1666. There was a rival theory that menstruation was caused by fermentation in the blood at certain times, e.g. Willis, p. 625.
27. Bartholin, p. 67.
28. Paré, p. 890.
29. Sadler, p. 10.
30. Paré, p. 910.
31. Dr Chamberlain, p. 63.
32. Willis, pp. 625–6.
33. Harvey, p. 504.
34. Mauriceau I, p. 324.
35. P. Portal, *The complete practice of men and women midwives* (1763) p. 249.
36. Sharp, p. 112.
37. Crooke, p. 193.
38. McMath, pp. 31–2.
39. Aristotle I, pp. 33–4.
40. As early as 1564 however Arantius had concluded from his dissection of a pregnant woman killed in an accident that the maternal and foetal bloodstreams are not continuous with one another, Needham pp. 86–7.
41. Dionis, p. 53.
42. Mauriceau I, pp. 167–8.
43. Pechey II, p. 89.
44. Mauriceau I, p. 256.
45. Raynald, f.42r.
46. McMath, p. 140.
47. Pechey II, p. 104.
48. Harvey, pp. 490–3.
49. Mauriceau I, p. 39.
50. Willughby, pp. 14–16.
51. Mauriceau I, pp. 142–5, 193.
52. Barret, pp. 37–8.
53. Mauriceau I, p. 323.
54. Giffard, p. 60.

## Chapter Seven Diagnosis of Pregnancy and Ante-natal Regimen

1. Pechey II, pp. 55–6. It was usual for a panel of matrons to examine female felons who had pleaded their belly, and according to their verdict the execution either proceeded or was stayed until after the delivery.
2. Sharp, p. 102.
3. Mauriceau I, p. 23.
4. Guillemeau, p. 109.
5. Raynald, f.141r-v.
6. Culpeper, p. 128.
7. Mauriceau I, p. 43.
8. Barret, p. 65.
9. Sudell, pp. 85–7.
10. Pechey II, pp. 54–5.
11. Aristotle I, p. 40.
12. Barret, pp. 60–61.
13. J. Oliver, *A present to be given to teeming women* (1688), the epistle to the reader.

14. W. Sermon, *The ladies companion, or the English midwife* (1671) p. 39.

15. This was the reason given for the Church prohibition of coitus during pregnancy, Noonan, p. 17. According to de Venette however, the French at any rate did not pay much attention to this rule.

16. Guillemeau, pp. 23–4.

17. Aristotle I, p. 43.

18. Dionis also mentions this custom of routine bleeding, though other authors do not, so perhaps it was a custom more common among Frenchwomen.

19. Anon, *A rich closet of physical secrets* (1652), p. 6. None of the practitioner authors suggests this, since they knew nothing could grow to the child anyway.

20. Guillemeau, p. 21.

21. Sharp, p. 103.

22. Maubray, pp. 62–3.

23. Mauriceau I, p. 231.

24. [Thomas Lewis], *Seasonable considerations on the indecent and dangerous custom of burying in churches and churchyards* (1721) p. 57.

25. Dr Chamberlain, pp. 92–3.

26. Aristotle I, p. 91.

27. Rueff, p. 2, second part.

28. G. Williams, *The age of agony: the art of healing c.1700–1800* (Constable, London, 1975) pp. 35–9.

## Chapter Eight Pregnancy Prevention and Promotion

1. J.T. Noonan, *Contraception* (Harvard UP, Cambridge, Mass., 1965) pp. 210–11.

2. The lines of thought in this chapter owe much to the stimulus of T.R. Forbes, *The midwife and the witch* (Yale UP, New Haven and London, 1966) and to Angus Maclaren, *Birth control in nineteenth century England* (Croom Helm, London 1978).

3. Raynald, the prologue.

4. Rueff, pp. 178–9.

5. Mauriceau II, p. 33.

6. Aristotle II, pp. 12–13.

7. Pechey I, p. 142.

8. Riverius, p. 403.

9. Sadler, p. 143.

10. Willughby, pp. 244–5.

11. Southampton Record Office, *Diary of John Casaubon 1674–1690*, p. 8.

12. T. Brugis, *Vade mecum*, 2nd edn (1653) the preface.

13. Rueff, pp. 59–61.

14. M. Mauquest de la Motte, *A general treatise of midwifery* (1724) p. 65.

15. F.G. Emmison, *Elizabethan life: morals and the Church courts* (Essex Record Office, Chelmsford, 1973) p. 41; Cheshire Consistory Court Records (EDC 5/1667/13). Reference kindly supplied by Mr David Harley.

16. T.R. Forbes, 'Regulation of midwives in the sixteenth and seventeenth centuries', *Med. Hist.* no. 8 (1964) pp. 235–44.

17. *Trials for adultery . . . being select trials at Doctors Commons . . . from the year 1760, to the present time* vol. 3, (1777) pp. 4–5.

18. Bartholin, p. 72.

19. Culpeper, p. 84.

20. Barrough, p. 158.

21. The source of our knowledge is libertine literature of the period, and personal papers.

22. Dionis, p. 365.

23. See Dorothy MacLaren, 'Fertility, infant mortality and breast feeding in the seventeenth century' *Med. Hist.* no. 22 (1978) pp. 378–96, and the same author's 'Nature's contraceptive. Wet nursing and prolonged lactation: the case of Chesham, Buckinghamshire 1578–1601' *Med. Hist.* no. 23 (1979) pp. 426–41.
24. Sharp, p. 31.
25. Sermon, pp. 11–13.
26. Riverius, p. 509.
27. Culpeper, p. 113.
28. Ibid. pp. 149–50.
29. Aristotle I, pp. 44–5.
30. Mauriceau I, pp. 135–6.

## Chapter Nine Gynaecology

1. Harvey, pp. 501–2.
2. Freind, p. 77.
3. Riverius, p. 404.
4. Sharp, p. 333.
5. Pechey I, p. 36.
6. Sudell, p. 12.
7. These fumigations were either wet or dry, and consisted of heating the liquid or solid medicaments over a brazier and passing the steam or smoke into the vagina through a pipe.
8. Riverius, pp. 411–2.
9. Pechey II, p. 221.
10. Ms Sloane 5, f.163v–164r.
11. C.R., p. 211.
12. Sharp, p. 62.
13. Riverius, p. 422.
14. Maubray, p. 402.
15. e.g. Willis, p. 632.
16. Pechey I, p. 67.
17. Willis, p. 629.
18. Pechey II, p. 235.
19. Dr Chamberlain, p. 60.
20. Pechey I, p. 4.
21. H. van Roonhuyse, *Medico-chirurgical observations* (1676) p. 73.
22. Dr Chamberlain, p. 61.
23. Harvey, p. 502.
24. C.R., p. 242.
25. Barrough, p. 151.
26. R. Hunter and I. Macalpine, *Three hundred years of psychiatry 1535–1860* (OUP, London, 1963) pp. 118, 133.
27. Sadler, p. 72.
28. Pechey I, p. 9.
29. Riverius, p. 427.
30. Willughby, p. 252.
31. Riverius, p. 501.
32. McMath, p. 271.
33. Sharp, pp. 39–40.
34. Riverius, p. 400.
35. Sudell, p. 10.
36. Maubray, p. 43.
37. Harvey, quoted in Hunter and Macalpine, p. 132.

38. Dr Chamberlain, p. 69.
39. Riverius, pp. 417–20.
40. Ibid., p. 413.
41. N. de Blegny, *New and curious observations on the art of curing the venereal disease* (1676) pp. 52–4.
42. Riverius, p. 492.
43. Sadler, p. 94.
44. Pechey II, p. 186.
45. Brockbank and Kenworthy (eds.), *The diary of Richard Kay . . .* , pp. 134–51 passim. I am much obliged to Dr T.H. Fahy for drawing my attention to this case.
46. Riverius, p. 493.

## Chapter Ten Normal Childbirth

1. Grantley Dick-Read, *Revelation of childbirth* (Heinemann, London, 1942).
2. C. White, *A treatise on the management of pregnant and lying-in women* (1773).
3. Jonas, f.7v.
4. Ibid., f.21r-v.
5. Mauriceau I, p. 180.
6. Willughby, p. 54.
7. J. Blunt, *Man-midwifery dissected* (1793) p. 28.
8. Dionis, p. 166.
9. Willis, p. 631.
10. Pechey II, p. 121.
11. Sudell, p. 62.
12. Sharp, pp. 199–200, Sermon, pp. 101–2.
13. Jonas, f.20v. This phrase does not appear in *De partu hominis* and was obviously not in the German original of that work, but was inserted by Jonas from his own knowledge by way of explanation.
14. Aristotle II, p. 50.
15. It seems that this method, though mentioned by several seventeenth-century authors, either was never very much used or fell into desuetude at a later date, so that when it was advocated in the nineteenth century by Credé it was taken to be his invention and became known as 'Credé's maneouvre'.
16. J. Harvie, *Practical directions showing a method of preserving the perineum in birth etc.* (1767), quoted in H. Thoms, *Classical contributions to obstetrics and gynecology* (Charles C. Thomas, Springfield, Ill., 1935) p. 135.
17. Maubray, p. 224.
18. H. van Deventer, *The art of midwifery improv'd* (1716) pp. 139–41.
19. Read, p. 561.
20. Chapman, pp. 132–3.
21. Barret, p. 13.
22. Sharp, p. 212.
23. Dionis, p. 285.
24. Chapman, p. 259.
25. Mauriceau II, pp. 292–3.
26. van Roonhuyse, p. 75.
27. Pechey II, pp. 128–9.
28. C.R., pp. 129–30.
29. Mauriceau II, p. 301.
30. Dionis, p. 287.
31. However some mothers made heroic efforts to nurse their children. Mauriceau stated that some had such severely cracked nipples that in the end the nipple was 'quite taken off' from the breast, but he gave directions for re-forming the

nipples using nipple-shields so that the mother could nurse again, Mauriceau I, p. 349.

32. C.R., pp. 21–2.
33. Wolveridge, p. 140.
34. Ibid., p. 145.
35. Ibid., p. 144.
36. *A rich closet of physical secrets*, p. 19.
37. Maubray, p. 333.
38. C.R., p. 21.
39. Mauriceau I, p. 366. The idea that colostrum was good for the baby, though taken up by Cadogan in his *Essay on nursing* (1748), had apparently had little impact by 1773, see C. White, p. 12.
40. J. Guillemeau, *The nursing of children* (1612) p. 18. Five days, during which the baby had a wet-nurse, was the time lapse before the mother attempted to nurse in the account given of the birth of judge Sewell of Boston in 1677 in H. Thoms, *Our obstetric heritage* (Shoe String Press Inc. Connecticut, 1960) p. 11.
41. Sharp p. 234.
42. Maubray pp. 333–4.
43. Willughby pp. 136–7.

## Chapter Eleven The Management of Obstetric Complications

1. Mauriceau I, p. 215.
2. Sermon, p. 120.
3. Willughby, p. 60.
4. Such a stone was kept in the custody of the Dean's wife at Canterbury for the use of women in difficult labour, Forbes, *The midwife and the witch*, p. 67.
5. Harvey, p. 488.
6. Willughby, p. 26.
7. Ibid., p. 158.
8. Chapman, pp. 135–6.
9. Giffard, p. 152.
10. Pechey I, pp. 144–5.
11. Read, p. 562.
12. Pechey, II pp. 142–3.
13. Willughby, p. 324.
14. Maubray, p. 246.
15. Jonas, f.40v.
16. Willughby, p. 54.
17. Dr Chamberlain, p. 149.
18. de Venette, p. 27.
19. A case of surgical delivery is described in detail by Guillemeau, pp. 107–10.
20. Harvey, pp. 492–3.
21. Willughby, p. 27.
22. Ibid., p. 187.
23. Portal, p. 264.
24. Chapman, p. 141.
25. Mauriceau I, pp. 306–7.
26. Willughby, pp. 199–201.

## Chapter Twelve 'The Manuall Practize' — Operative Delivery

1. Jonas, f.51r-52v.

2. There is however an account of a labourer making iron hooks with which he delivered his wife of a dead child on the midwife's instructions at Myddle in the seventeenth century in D.G. Hey, *An English rural community. Myddle under the Tudors and Stuarts* (Leicester UP, 1974) p. 183.
3. Willughby, p. 151.
4. Mauriceau I, the translator to the reader.
5. Sermon, p. 141.
6. Willughby, pp. 87–8.
7. Mauriceau I, p. 205.
8. Read, p. 557.
9. Willughby, p. 57.
10. McMath, p. 179.
11. Mauriceau I, pp. 240–1.
12. Guillemeau p. 140.
13. Willughby, p. 192.
14. Read, p. 589.
15. J.H. Young, *Caesarean section: the history and development of the operation from the earliest times* (H.K. Lewis, London, 1944) p. 22.
16. F. Rousset, *Traité nouveau de l'hysterotomotokie ou enfantement caesarien* (1581) p. 12.
17. Guillemeau, pp. 187–8.
18. Paré, p. 923.
19. Mauriceau I, pp. 276–7.
20. Willughby, p. 101.
21. Rousset, pp. 34–5, 46–7.
22. Mauriceau I, p. 278.
23. Young, p. 54.
24. Sharp, p. 197.
25. van Roonhuyse, p. 16.
26. Mr David Harley of the Wellcome Unit for the History of Medicine, Oxford, in the course of some unpublished research, has found that at least in Lancashire and Cheshire there were rather more of these literate midwives of higher social standing than has been hitherto realised. So far as he is aware however they were not *professionally* superior to those of lower socio-economic status, and learned their art in the traditional manner from other midwives, sometimes relatives. He has found only one who certainly possessed a midwifery textbook, but in view of the rarity of wills and inventories relating to the estates of women this could be viewed as an important positive indication. .
27. Willughby, pp. 130–1.
28. Ibid., pp. 125–6.
29. Read, pp. 574–5.
30. Willughby, p. 164.
31. Ibid., pp. 154–5.
32. Mauriceau II, the translator to the reader.
33. See J.H. Aveling, *The Chamberlens and the midwifery forceps* (Churchill, London, 1882) and W. Radcliffe, *The secret instrument* (Heinemann, London, 1947).
34. Chapman, preface p. xxi.

## Chapter Thirteen Two Centuries of Obstetric Change Reviewed

1. Such a dried caul in a box was shown to Miss S.J. MacPherson quite recently on a visit to a Women's Institute.
2. This idea persisted even into the present century, as some of the letters sent to Dr Marie Stopes reveal; R. Hall(ed.), *Dear Dr. Stopes* (André Deutsch, London, 1978).
3. A woman at Chesterfield in Derbyshire in 1646 had several midwives to assist her;

'one of them thrust up her hand, and made great struggling in her body; at the taking of it forth, her hand was all over bloody, and this midwife made great vaunts of her skil, and doings, and said, That the child did stick to the woman's back, but that shee had removed it' Willughby, p. 7.

## Appendix Maternal Mortality: Somes Notes on the Willughby Cases

1. Blunt, p. 176.
2. A. Eccles, 'Obstetrics in the 17th and 18th centuries and its implications for maternal and infant mortality' *Bull. Soc. Social Hist. Med.*, no. 20 (1977) pp. 8–11. Summary only.
3. Very few parish registers except those within the London bills of mortality record the burials of stillborn children.
4. Cumbria County Record Office (Carlisle) D/Lons/L A1/4 Sir John Lowther's diary. I am much indebted to Dr Colin Phillips for drawing my attention to this interesting case.
5. Willughby, p. 205.
6. Ibid., pp. 124–5.
7. Ibid., p. 83.
8. C. Wells, 'Ancient obstetric hazards and female mortality' *Bull. NY Acad. Med.*, no. 51 (1975) pp. 1235–49.
9. The very words 'rickets' and 'rachitis' were coined in the seventeenth century, and rickets is one of the few causes of death listed in the bills of mortality. Glisson in 1651 stated that it was 'absolutely a new Disease, and never described by any of the Ancient or Modern Writers in their practical Books which are extant at this day, of the Diseases of Infants', Glisson, p. 3.
10. Willughby, pp. 81–2.
11. Ibid., pp. 112–14.
12. The story is well known of Hugh Chamberlen's attempt to sell the secret of the forceps to Mauriceau, and of his total failure to deliver the rachitic dwarf he was given to demonstrate on, Radcliffe, pp. 21–4.
13. Willughby, pp. 321–4.
14. Ibid., pp. 114–15.
15. Ibid., p. 111.
16. Ibid., p. 214.
17. Ibid., pp. 210–11.
18. Ibid., p. 217.
19. Willis, pp. 626–7.
20. Willughby, p. 222.
21. Ibid., p. 117.
22. Ibid., p. 155.

# Index